The Child and Adolescent Psychotherapy Treatment Planner

The Child and Adolescent Psychotherapy Treatment Planner

Arthur E. Jongsma

L. Mark Peterson

William P. McInnis

JOHN WILEY & SONS, INC.

New York • Chichester • Brisbane • Toronto • Singapore

Copyright © 1996 by Arthur E. Jongsma, Jr., L. Mark Peterson, and William P. McInnis

Published by John Wiley & Sons, Inc.

Library of Congress Cataloging-in-Publication Data

Jongsma, Arthur E., 1943–
    The child and adolescent psychotherapy treatment planner / by
Arthur E. Jongsma, L. Mark Peterson, William P. McInnis.
      p.   cm.
    Includes bibliographical references (p.).
    ISBN 0-471-15647-7 (pbk. : alk. paper)
    1. Child psychotherapy.   2. Adolescent psychotherapy.
I. Peterson, L. Mark. II. McInnis, William P. III. Title.
RJ504.J66   1996
618.92'8914—dc20   96-16093
                                          CIP

To our wives: Judy, Cherry, and Lynn.
We reach our long-term goals
only due to your faithful interventions
of love and encouragement.

PREFACE

The enthusiastic response to *The Complete Psychotherapy Treatment Planner* (A. E. Jongsma and L. M. Peterson, Wiley, 1995) and its electronic companion, *TheraScribe* (Wiley, 1996), has highlighted the need for tools that can help clinicians cope with the ever-increasing paperwork in clinical practice. We are delighted that our experience in developing behaviorally oriented treatment plans has been of benefit to the thousands of psychologists, psychiatrists, social workers, and counselors who embraced the original planner. Many of our colleagues who use the adult *Planner* urged us to develop a counterpart that deals with treatment planning for children and teenagers.

So we are pleased to introduce *The Child and Adolescent Psychotherapy Treatment Planner*. This new *Planner* offers prewritten behavioral definitions, objectives, goals, and interventions for dozens of disorders encountered in younger clients. Like its predecessor (which focused primarily on adult disorders), *The Child and Adolescent Planner* is designed to stimulate thought, ease the paperwork crunch, and help clinicians develop treatment plans that meet the needs of managed care reviewers.

Although *The Child and Adolescent Planner* follows the same format as the adult planner, we have made one slight adjustment in emphasis. Since many people commented on how helpful they found the suggestions for therapeutic interventions in the original planner, we have expanded the interventions featured in this book. As with the adult edition, these interventions are eclectic in origin, spanning the range from cognitive, behavioral, dynamic, familial, pharmacological, educational, and didactic to bibliotherapeutic and assessment oriented. It is our hope that *The Child and Adolescent Planner* will serve as a treatment consultant, offering a wide variety of therapeutic ideas for your clinical consideration and streamlining the planning process.

Neither *The Child and Adolescent Psychotherapy Treatment Planner* nor the original adult edition would have been possible without the support of a terrific cadre of colleagues. We would like to offer our thanks to the individuals who reviewed the manuscript and offered many insightful suggestions. Susan Zonnebelt-Smeenge, Ed.D., a psychologist who specializes in treatment of anorexia and bulimia, gave valuable feedback on the eating disorders chapter. Patricia Edwards, M.A., C.C.C., consulted on the speech and language disorders section. David Berghuis, M.A., a clinician who works with developmentally disabled clients, offered suggestions regarding objectives and interventions for mentally retarded clients. We are grateful to each of these professionals for their candid and crucial advice.

No manuscript finds its way to a publisher without the cooperative efforts and support of a variety of talented people. This project was word-processed endlessly by Judy Jongsma, Kendra van Elst, Marcia Berends, and Cherry Peterson. We would like to thank each of these troupers for their perseverance and help in getting the book completed when it needed to be done yesterday.

No book finds its way into print without the guidance and support of an editor. Some editors just crank out books that are like flavorless quarter-pounders with cheese. Kelly Franklin, of John Wiley & Sons, settles for no less than chateaubriand. She cracked the whip at deadline time, warmly encouraged us at the frustrating stages, and judiciously brandished a sharply honed pencil when the project was near completion. Kelly, you are the best!

Finally, no writing reaches completion without the sacrifice of the authors' discretionary time. Our wives and children have seen less of us as we gave ourselves to this effort over the last few months. We appreciate their understanding and extend our gratitude for their loving support.

Arthur E. Jongsma, Jr., Ph.D.
L. Mark Peterson, M.S.W.
William P. McInnis, Psy.D.

CONTENTS

INTRODUCTION

Since the early 1960s, formalized treatment planning has gradually become a vital aspect of the entire health care delivery system, whether it is treatment related to physical health, mental health, child welfare, or substance abuse. What started in the medical sector in the 1960s spread into the mental health sector in the 1970s as clinics, psychiatric hospitals, agencies, and so on, began to seek accreditation from bodies such as the Joint Commission on Accreditation of Healthcare Organizations (JCAHO) to qualify for third-party reimbursements. For most treatment providers to achieve accreditation, they had to begin developing and strengthening their documentation skills in the area of treatment planning. Previously, most mental health and substance abuse treatment providers had, at best, a "bare-bones" plan that looked similar for most of the individuals they treated. As a result, clients were uncertain about what they were trying to attain in mental health treatment. Goals were vague, objectives were nonexistent, and interventions were applied equally to all clients. Outcome data were not measurable, and neither the treatment provider nor the client knew exactly when treatment was complete. The initial development of rudimentary treatment plans made inroads toward addressing some of these issues.

With the advent of managed care in the 1980s, treatment planning has taken on even more importance. Managed care systems *insist* that clinicians move rapidly from assessment of the problem to the formulation and implementation of the treatment plan. The goal of most managed care companies is to expedite the treatment process by prompting the client and treatment provider to focus on identifying and changing behavioral problems as quickly as possible. Treatment plans must be specific as to the problems and interventions, individualized to meet the client's needs and goals, and measurable in terms of setting milestones that can be used to chart the client's progress. Pressure from third-party payers, accrediting agencies, and other outside parties has therefore increased the need for clinicians to produce effective, high-quality treatment plans in a short time frame. However, many mental health providers have little experience in treatment plan development. Our purpose in writing this book is to clarify, simplify, and accelerate the treatment planning process.

TREATMENT PLAN UTILITY

Detailed written treatment plans can benefit not only the client, therapist, treatment team, insurance community, and treatment agency, but also the overall psychotherapy profession. The client is served by a written plan because it stipulates the issues that are the focus of the treatment process. It is very easy for both provider and client to lose sight of what the issues were that brought the client into therapy. The treatment plan is a guide that structures the focus of the therapeutic contract. Since issues can change as therapy progresses, the treatment plan must be viewed as a dynamic document that can and must be updated to reflect any major change of problem, definition, goal, objective, or intervention.

Clients and therapists benefit from the treatment plan, which forces both to think about therapy outcomes. Behaviorally stated, measurable objectives clearly focus the treatment endeavor. Clients no longer have to wonder what therapy is trying to accomplish. Clear objectives also allow the client to channel effort into specific changes that will lead to the long-term goal of problem resolution. Therapy is no longer a vague contract to just talk honestly and openly about emotions and cognitions until the client feels better. Both client and therapist are concentrating on specifically stated objectives using specific interventions.

Providers are aided by treatment plans because they are forced to think analytically and critically about therapeutic interventions that are best suited for objective attainment for the client. Therapists were traditionally trained to "follow the client," but now a formalized plan is the guide to the treatment process. The therapist must give advance attention to the technique, approach, assignment, or cathartic target that will form the basis for interventions.

Clinicians benefit from clear documentation of treatment because it provides a measure of added protection from possible client litigation. Malpractice suits are increasing in frequency and insurance premiums are soaring. The first line of defense against allegations is a complete clinical record detailing the treatment process. A written, individualized, formal treatment plan that is the guideline for the therapeutic process, that has been reviewed and signed by the client, and that is coupled with problem-oriented progress notes is a powerful defense against exaggerated or false claims.

A well-crafted treatment plan that clearly stipulates presenting problems and intervention strategies facilitates the treatment process carried out by team members in inpatient, residential, or intensive outpatient settings. Good communication between team members about what approach is being implemented and who is responsible for which intervention is critical. Team meetings to discuss client treatment used to be the only source of interaction between providers; often, therapeutic conclusions or assignments were not recorded. Now, a thorough treatment plan stipulates in writing the details of objectives and the varied interventions (pharmacologic, milieu, group therapy, didactic, recreational, individual therapy, and so on) and who will implement them.

Every treatment agency or institution is constantly looking for ways to increase the quality and uniformity of the documentation in the clinical record. A standardized, written treatment plan with problem definitions, goals, objectives, and interventions in every client's file enhances that uniformity of documentation. This uniformity eases the task of record reviewers inside and outside the agency. Outside reviewers, such as JCAHO, insist on documentation that clearly outlines assessment, treatment, progress, and discharge status.

The demand for accountability from third-party payers and health maintenance organizations (HMOs) is partially satisfied by a written treatment plan and complete progress notes. More and more managed care systems are demanding a structured therapeutic contract that has measurable objectives and explicit interventions. Clinicians cannot avoid this move toward being accountable to those outside the treatment process.

The psychotherapy profession stands to benefit from the use of more precise, measurable objectives to evaluate success in mental health treatment. With the advent of detailed treatment plans, outcome data can be more easily collected for interventions that are effective in achieving specific goals.

HOW TO DEVELOP A TREATMENT PLAN

The process of developing a treatment plan involves a logical series of steps that build on each other much like constructing a house. The foundation of any effective treatment plan is the data gathered in a thorough biopsychosocial assessment. As the client presents himself or herself for treatment, the clinician must sensitively listen to and understand what the client struggles with in terms of family-of-origin issues, current stressors, emotional status, social network, physical health, coping skills, interpersonal conflicts, self-esteem, and so on. Assessment data may be gathered from a social history, physical exam, clinical interview, psychological testing, or contact with a client's significant others. The integration of the data by the clinician or the multidisciplinary treatment team members is critical for understanding the client, as is an awareness of the basis of the client's struggle. We have identified six specific steps for developing an effective treatment plan based on the assessment data.

Step One: Problem Selection

Although the client may discuss a variety of issues during the assessment, the clinician must ferret out the most significant problems on which to focus the treatment process. Usually a *primary* problem will surface, and *secondary* problems may also be evident. Some *other* problems may have to be set aside as not urgent enough to require treatment at this time. An effective treatment plan can only deal with a few selected problems or treatment will lose its direction. This *Planner* offers twenty-nine problems from which to select those that most accurately represent your client's presenting issues.

As the problems to be selected become clear to the clinician or the treatment team, it is important to include opinions from the client as to his or her prioritization of issues for which help is being sought. A client's motivation to participate in and cooperate with the treatment process depends, to some extent, on the degree to which treatment addresses his or her greatest needs.

Step Two: Problem Definition

Each individual client presents with unique nuances as to how a problem behaviorally reveals itself in his or her life. Therefore, each problem that is selected for treatment focus requires a specific definition about how it is evidenced in the particular client. The symptom pattern should be associated with diagnostic criteria and codes such as those found in the *Diagnostic and Statistical Manual* or the *International Classification of Diseases*. The *Planner,* following the pattern established by DSM-IV, offers such behaviorally specific definition statements to choose from or to serve as a model for your own personally crafted statements. You will find several behavior symptoms or syndromes listed that may characterize one of the twenty-nine presenting problems.

Step Three: Goal Development

The next step in treatment plan development is that of setting broad goals for the resolution of the target problem. These statements need not be crafted in measurable terms but can be global, long-term goals that indicate a desired positive outcome to the treatment procedures. The *Planner* suggests several possible goal statements for each problem, but one statement is all that is required in a treatment plan.

Step Four: Objective Construction

In contrast to long-term goals, objectives must be stated in behaviorally measurable language. It must be clear when the client has achieved the established objectives; therefore, vague, subjective objectives are not acceptable. Review agencies (e.g., JCAHO), HMOs, and managed care organizations insist that psychological treatment outcome be measurable. The objectives presented in this *Planner* are designed to meet this demand for accountability. Numerous alternatives are presented to allow construction of a variety of treatment plan possibilities for the same presenting problem. The clinician must exercise professional judgment as to which objectives are most appropriate for a given client.

Each objective should be developed as a step toward attaining the broad treatment goal. In essence, objectives can be thought of as a series of steps that, when completed, will result in the achievement of the long-term goal. There should be at least two objectives for each problem, but the clinician may construct as many as are necessary for goal achievement. Target attainment dates should be listed for each objective. New objectives should be added to the plan as the individual's treatment progresses. When all the necessary objectives have been achieved, the client should have resolved the target problem successfully.

Step Five: Intervention Creation

Interventions are the actions of the clinician designed to help the client complete the objectives. There should be at least one intervention for every objective. If the client does not accomplish the objective after the initial intervention, new interventions should be added to the plan.

Interventions should be selected on the basis of the client's needs and the treatment provider's full therapeutic repertoire. This *Planner* contains interventions from a broad range of therapeutic approaches, including cognitive, dynamic, behavioral, pharmacologic, family-oriented, and solution-focused brief therapy. Other interventions may be written by the provider to reflect his or her own training and experience. The addition of new problems, definitions, goals, objectives, and interventions to those found in the *Planner* is encouraged because doing so adds to the database for future reference and use.

Some suggested interventions listed in the *Planner* refer to specific books that can be assigned to the client for adjunctive bibliotherapy. Appendix A contains a full bibliographic reference list of these materials. The books are arranged under each problem for which they are appropriate as assigned reading for clients. When a book is used as part of an intervention plan, it should be reviewed with the client after it is read, enhancing the application of the content of the book to the specific client's circumstances. For further information about self-help books, mental health professionals may wish to consult *The Authoritative Guide to Self-Help Books* (1994) by Santrock, Minnett, and Campbell (available from The Guilford Press, New York).

Assigning an intervention to a specific provider is most relevant if the client is being treated by a team in an inpatient, residential, or intensive outpatient setting. Within these settings, personnel other than the primary clinician may be responsible for implementing a specific intervention. Review agencies require that the responsible provider's name be stipulated for every intervention.

Step Six: Diagnosis Determination

The determination of an appropriate diagnosis is based on an evaluation of the client's complete clinical presentation. The clinician must compare the behavioral, cognitive, emotional, and interpersonal symptoms that the client presents to the criteria for diagnosis of a mental illness condition as described in DSM-IV. The issue of differential diagnosis is admittedly a difficult one that research has shown to have rather low inter-rater reliability. Psychologists have also been trained to think more in terms of maladaptive behavior than in disease labels. In spite of these factors, diagnosis is a reality that exists in the world of mental health care and it is a necessity for third-party reimbursement. (However, recently, managed care agencies are more interested in behavioral indices that are exhibited by the client than in the actual diagnosis.) It is the clinician's thorough knowledge of DSM-IV criteria and a complete understanding of the client assessment data that contribute to the most reliable, valid diagnosis. An accurate assessment of behavioral indicators will also contribute to more effective treatment planning.

HOW TO USE THIS PLANNER

Our experience has taught us that learning the skills of effective treatment plan writing can be a tedious and difficult process for many clinicians. It is more stressful to try to develop this expertise when under the pressure of increased client load and short time frames placed on clinicians today by managed care systems. The documentation demands can be overwhelming when we must move quickly from assessment to treatment plan to progress notes. In the process, we must be very specific about how and when objectives can be achieved, and how progress is exhibited in each client. *The Child and Adolescent Psychotherapy Treatment Planner* was developed as a tool to aid clinicians in writing a treatment plan in a rapid manner that is clear, specific, and highly individualized according to the following progression:

1. Choose one presenting problem (Step One) you have identified through your assessment process. Locate the corresponding page number for that problem in the *Planner*'s table of contents.
2. Select two or three of the listed behavioral definitions (Step Two) and record them in the appropriate section on your treatment plan form. Feel free to add your own defining statement if you determine that your client's behavioral manifestation of the identified problem is not listed. (Note that while our design for treatment planning is vertical, it will work equally well on plan forms formatted horizontally.)
3. Select a single long-term goal (Step Three) and again write the selection, exactly as it is written in the *Planner* or in some appropriately modified form, in the corresponding area of your own form.
4. Review the listed objectives for this problem and select the ones that you judge to be clinically indicated for your client (Step Four). Remember, it is recommended that you select at least two objectives for each problem. Add a target date or the number of sessions allocated for the attainment of each objective.
5. Choose relevant interventions (Step Five). The *Planner* offers suggested interventions related to each objective in the parentheses following the objective statement. But do not limit yourself to those interventions. The entire list is eclectic and may offer options that are more tailored to your theoretical approach or preferred way of working with clients. Also, just as with definitions, goals, and objectives, there is space allowed for you to enter your own interventions into the *Planner*. This allows you to refer to these entries when you create a plan around this prob-

lem in the future. You will have to assign responsibility to a specific person for implementation of each intervention if the treatment is being carried out by a multidisciplinary team.

6. Several DSM-IV diagnoses are listed at the end of each chapter that are commonly associated with a client who has this problem. These diagnoses are meant to be suggestions for clinical consideration. Select a diagnosis listed or assign a more appropriate choice from the DSM-IV (Step Six).

Note: To accommodate those practitioners who tend to plan treatment in terms of diagnostic labels rather than presenting problems, Appendix B lists all of the DSM-IV diagnoses that have been presented in the various presenting problem chapters as suggestions for consideration. Each diagnosis is followed by the presenting problem that has been associated with that diagnosis. The provider may look up the presenting problems for a selected diagnosis to review definitions, goals, objectives, and interventions that may be appropriate for their clients with that diagnosis.

Congratulations! You should now have a complete, individualized treatment plan that is ready for immediate implementation and presentation to the client. It should resemble the format of the sample plan presented on the facing page.

A FINAL NOTE

One important aspect of effective treatment planning is that each plan should be tailored to the individual client's problems and needs. Treatment plans should not be mass-produced, even if clients have similar problems. The individual's strengths and weaknesses, unique stressors, social network, family circumstances, and symptom patterns *must* be considered in developing a treatment strategy. Drawing upon our own years of clinical experience, we have put together a variety of treatment choices. These statements can be combined in thousands of permutations to develop detailed treatment plans. Relying on their own good judgment, clinicians can easily select the statements that are appropriate for the individuals they are treating. In addition, we encourage readers to add their own definitions, goals, objectives, and interventions to the existing samples. It is our hope that *The Child and Adolescent Psychotherapy Treatment Planner* will promote effective, creative treatment planning—a process that will ultimately benefit the client, clinician, and mental health community.

SAMPLE TREATMENT PLAN

Problem: PHYSICAL ABUSE VICTIM

Definitions: Confirmed self-report or account by others of the client being assaulted (e.g., hit, burned, kicked, slapped, or tortured) by an older person.

Pronounced disturbance of mood and affect (i.e., frequent and prolonged periods of depression, irritability, anxiety, and apathetic withdrawal).

Goals: Terminate physical abuse of the client.

Resolve the client's feelings of fear and depression while improving communication and the boundaries of respect within the family.

Objectives	Interventions
1. Identify the nature, frequency, and duration of the abuse (6/22/96).	1. Actively build the level of trust with the client in individual sessions through consistent eye contact, active listening, unconditional positive regard, and warm acceptance to help increase the client's ability to identify and express feelings.
2. Identify and express the feelings connected to the abuse (7/12/96).	1. Explore, encourage, and support the client in verbally expressing and clarifying feelings associated with the abuse.
	2. Utilize individual play therapy sessions to provide the client with the opportunity to express and work through feelings of hurt, fear, and anger related to the abuse.

(Continued)

3. Stabilize the mood and decrease the emotional intensity connected to the abuse (7/26/96).

1. Hold a family session where the perpetrator apologizes to the client and/or other family member(s) for the abuse.

4. Increase self-esteem as evidenced by more frequent positive self-descriptive statements, improved eye contact, and a stronger voice (8/26/96).

1. Assist the client in identifying a basis for self-worth by reviewing his/her talents, importance to others, and intrinsic spiritual value.

2. Reinforce positive statements made about the self and the future.

Diagnosis: 300.4   Dysthymic Disorder
                 V61.21   Physical Abuse of Child, 995.54 Victim

SUMMARY

Our experience has taught us that learning the skills of effective treatment plan writing can be a tedious and difficult process for many clinicians. It is more stressful to try to develop this expertise when under the pressure of the increased client loads and short time frames placed on clinicians today by managed care systems. The documentation demands can be overwhelming when we must move quickly from assessment to treatment plan to progress notes. In the process we must be very specific about how and when objectives can be achieved and exhibited in each individual client. This *Planner* was developed as a tool to aid clinicians in writing treatment plans in a rapid manner that is clear, specific, and highly individualized. We have put together a variety of choices to allow for thousands of potential combinations of statements that join to make a completed plan for treatment. Clinicians with their good judgment can easily select statements that are appropriate for the individuals they are treating. Each statement can be modified as necessary to more directly apply to a specific individual client. Finally, we believe from our experience that the *Planner* method of treatment plan construction is helpful in that it stimulates creative thoughts by clinicians. New ideas for all components of a treatment plan may come to mind as the *Planner* statements are reviewed. Clinicians can add to the *Planner* by writing in new definitions, goals, objectives, and interventions.

ANXIETY

BEHAVIORAL DEFINITIONS

1. Excessive anxiety, worry, or fear that markedly exceeds the level for the client's stage of development.
2. High level of motor tension such as restlessness, tiredness, shakiness, or muscle tension.
3. Autonomic hyperactivity such as rapid heartbeat, shortness of breath, dizziness, dry mouth, nausea, or diarrhea.
4. Hypervigilance such as feeling constantly on edge, concentration difficulties, trouble falling or staying asleep, and a general state of irritability.
5. A specific fear that has become generalized to cover a wide area and has reached the point where it significantly interferes with the client's and the family's daily life.
6. Excessive anxiety or worry due to a parent's threat of abandonment, overuse of guilt, denial of autonomy and status, friction between parents, or interference with physical activity.

__. _____
   _____
__. _____
   _____
__. _____
   _____

LONG-TERM GOALS

1. Reduce the overall frequency and intensity of the anxiety response so that daily functioning is not impaired.

2. Stabilize the anxiety level while increasing the ability to function on a daily basis.
3. Resolve the key issue that is the source of the anxiety or fear.
4. Reach the point where the client can interact with the world without excessive fear, worry, or anxiety.

__. _____

_____

__. _____

_____

__. _____

_____

SHORT-TERM OBJECTIVES

1. Develop a working relationship with the therapist in which the client openly shares thoughts and feelings. (1, 2)
2. Verbally identify fears, worries, and anxieties. (1, 2, 8, 9)
3. Implement positive self-talk to reduce or eliminate the anxiety. (1, 3, 4, 7)
4. Increase the coping behaviors of peer socialization, physical activity, and self-reassurance. (7, 10, 11, 13)
5. Increase participation in daily social and academic activities. (8, 11, 13, 14)

THERAPEUTIC INTERVENTIONS

1. Actively build the level of trust with the client in individual sessions through consistent eye contact, active listening, unconditional positive regard, and warm acceptance to help increase his/her ability to identify and express feelings.
2. Use a therapeutic game (Talking, Feeling, Doing* or The Ungame†) to expand the client's awareness of self and others.
3. Help the client develop reality-based cognitive messages that will increase self-confidence in coping with fears and anxieties.

_____

* Creative Therapeutics, Cresskill, New Jersey, 1973.
† The Ungame Co., Anaheim, California, 1984.

6. Develop and implement appropriate relaxation and diversion activities to decrease the level of anxiety. (7, 12, 14, 15)

7. Identify areas of conflict in the client's life. (5, 6, 12, 15)

8. The parents verbalize an understanding of the client's anxieties and fears. (16, 17, 18, 19)

9. The parents develop specific ways to empathically help the client with the anxiety and fear. (20, 21, 22, 23)

—. _____
    _____
—. _____
    _____
—. _____
    _____

4. Explore cognitive messages that mediate the anxiety response and retrain the client in adaptive cognitions.

5. Ask the client to develop a list of key past and present conflicts within the family and with peers. Process this list with the therapist.

6. Assist the client to become aware of key conflicts and start to work toward their resolution.

7. Help the client develop healthy self-talk as a means of handling the anxiety.

8. Use a narrative approach (Michael White)* in which the client writes out the story of his/her anxiety or fear and then acts out the story with the therapist to externalize the issues. Then work with the client to reach a resolution or develop an effective way to cope with the anxiety or fear.

9. Conduct play therapy sessions in which the client's anxieties, fears, and worries are explored and resolved.

10. Utilize an interpretive play interview method in which the therapist interviews the client to help express motivation and feelings. Then assist the client in making

* M. White and D. Epston, *Narrative Means to Therapeutic Ends* (New York: Norton, 1990).

a connection between fears or anxieties and unexpressed or unacceptable wishes or "bad" thoughts.

11. Encourage the parents to seek an experiential camp or weekend experience for the client that will focus on the issues of fears, taking risks, and building trust. Process the experience with the client and his/her parents.

12. Conduct sessions with a focus on anxiety-producing situations in which techniques of storytelling, drawing pictures, viewing photographs, and doing homework are used to reduce the level of anxiety or fear in the client.

13. Assist the client in developing anxiety-coping strategies (e.g., increased social involvement, contact with peers, physical exercise).

14. Advocate and encourage overthinking. Monitor weekly results and redirect as needed.

15. Use a mutual storytelling technique (by Richard Gardner)* in which the client tells his/her story. The therapist interprets the story for its underlying meaning and then tells

---

* R. Gardner, *Story Telling in Psychotherapy with Children* (New York: J. Aronson, 1993).

his/her own story using the same characters in a similar setting, but weaving into the story healthier adaptations to fear or anxiety and resolution of conflicts.

16. Educate the client's parents to increase their awareness and understanding of what fears and anxieties are developmentally normal for children or teens at each age.

17. Assign the client's parents to read books related to child development and parenting such as *Between Parent and Child / Teenager* (Ginott) or *How to Talk So Kids Will Listen and Listen So Kids Will Talk* (Faber and Mazlish).

18. Refer the client's parents to a parenting class or support group.

19. Work with the parents in family sessions to develop their skills in effectively handling the client's fears and anxieties with calm confidence rather than fearful reactivity.

20. Conduct family sessions in which the system is probed to determine the level of fear or anxiety that is present or to bring to the surface underlying conflicts.

21. Work in family sessions to resolve conflicts and to increase the family's level of healthy functioning.

22. Use a structural approach in the family session in which roles are adjusted to encourage the parents to work less and allow kids to be kids.

23. Conduct family sessions in which strategic directions that are designed to increase the physical freedom of the children and to adjust the parental control of the system are developed and given to the family.

___. _____

_____

___. _____

_____

___. _____

_____

DIAGNOSTIC SUGGESTIONS

Axis I: 300.02   Generalized Anxiety Disorder
300.00   Anxiety Disorder NOS
309.24   Adjustment Disorder With Anxiety
314.01   Attention-Deficit/Hyperactivity Disorder, Combined Type
309.21   Separation Anxiety Disorder

_____   _____

_____   _____

Axis II: 799.9   Diagnosis Deferred
V71.09   No Diagnosis

_____   _____

_____   _____

ATTENTION-DEFICIT/ HYPERACTIVITY DISORDER

BEHAVIORAL DEFINITIONS

1. Short attention span; difficulty sustaining attention on a consistent basis.
2. Susceptibility to distraction by extraneous stimuli.
3. Impression that he/she is not listening well.
4. Repeated failure to follow through on instructions or complete school assignments, chores, or job responsibilities in a timely manner.
5. Poor organizational skills as demonstrated by forgetfulness, inattention to details, and losing things necessary for tasks.
6. Hyperactivity as evidenced by a high energy level, restlessness, difficulty sitting still, or loud or excessive talking.
7. Impulsivity as evidenced by difficulty awaiting his/her turn in group situations, blurting out answers to questions before the questions have been completed, and frequent intrusions into others' personal business.
8. Frequent disruptive, aggressive, or negative attention-seeking behaviors.
9. Tendency to engage in careless or potentially dangerous activities.
10. Difficulty accepting responsibility for actions, projecting blame for problems onto others, and failing to learn from experience.
11. Low self-esteem and poor social skills.

—. _____

_____

—. _____

_____

—. _____

_____

LONG-TERM GOALS

1. Sustain attention and concentration for consistently longer periods of time.
2. Increase the frequency of on-task behaviors as manifested by regular completion of school assignments, chores, and work responsibilities.
3. Demonstrate marked improvement in impulse control as evidenced by a significant reduction in aggressive, disruptive, and negative attention-seeking behaviors.
4. Regularly take medication as prescribed to decrease impulsivity, hyperactivity, and distractibility.
5. The parents and/or teachers successfully utilize a reward system, contingency contract, or token economy to reinforce positive behaviors and deter negative behaviors.
6. The parents set firm, consistent limits and maintain appropriate parent-child boundaries.
7. Improve self-esteem as evidenced by an increase in positive self-statements and participation in extracurricular activities.
8. Maintain lasting peer friendships.

—. _____

_____

—. _____

_____

—. _____

_____

SHORT-TERM OBJECTIVES

1. Complete psychological testing to confirm the diagnosis of ADHD. (1, 2, 3)

2. Complete psychological testing to rule out emotional factors or learning disabilities as the basis for maladaptive behavior. (1, 2, 3)

3. Begin to take prescribed medication as directed by the physician. (4, 5)

4. Increase on-task behaviors as evidenced by greater completion of school assignments, chores, and work responsibilities. (7, 8, 9, 11, 28)

5. The parents develop and utilize an organized system to keep track of school assignments, chores, and work responsibilities. (7, 8, 9, 10)

6. Establish a routine schedule to help complete homework, chores, and household responsibilities. (8, 9, 10, 11, 12)

7. The parents and teachers reduce extraneous stimuli as much as possible when giving directions to the client. (6, 10, 11, 13)

8. The parents maintain communication with the school to increase the client's compliance with completion of school assignments. (9, 11)

THERAPEUTIC INTERVENTIONS

1. Arrange for psychological testing to confirm the presence of ADHD in the client.

2. Arrange for psychological testing to rule out emotional factors or learning disabilities as the basis for the client's maladaptive behavior.

3. Give feedback to the client and his/her family regarding psychological testing results.

4. Arrange for a medication evaluation for the client.

5. Monitor the client for compliance, side effects, and overall effectiveness of the medication. Consult with the prescribing physician at regular intervals.

6. Educate the client's parents and siblings about the symptoms of ADHD.

7. Assist the parents in developing and implementing an organizational system to increase the client's on-task behaviors and completion of school assignments, chores, or work responsibilities (e.g., use of calendars, charts, notebooks, and class syllabus).

8. Assist the parents in developing a routine schedule to increase the client's compliance with school, household, or work-related responsibilities.

9. Teachers utilize a *listening buddy* who sits next to the client in the classroom to quietly answer questions or repeat instructions. (10, 11)

10. Teachers schedule breaks between intensive instructional periods and alternate complex activities with less stressful activities to sustain the client's interest and attention. (11, 15, 19)

11. Teachers reinforce on-task behaviors, completion of school assignments, and good impulse control. (15, 17, 19)

12. Decrease motor activity as evidenced by the ability to sit still for longer periods of time. (5, 14, 17, 29)

13. The parents set firm limits and use natural, logical consequences to deter the client's impulsive behaviors. (6, 16, 17, 18, 20)

14. The parents identify and utilize a variety of effective reinforcers to increase positive behaviors. (15, 17, 21)

15. The parents increase praise and positive verbalizations toward the client. (6, 15, 17, 21)

16. The client and his/her parents comply with the implementation of a reward system or contingency contract. (17, 18, 20)

17. Reduce the frequency and severity of temper outbursts, acting out, and

9. Encourage the parents and teachers to maintain regular communication about the client's academic, behavioral, emotional, and social progress.

10. Teach the client more effective study skills (e.g., clear away distractions, study in quiet places, outline or underline important details, use a tape recorder, schedule breaks in studying).

11. Consult with his/her teachers to implement strategies to improve the client's school performance (e.g., sit in front of the class, use a prearranged signal to redirect the client back to the task, provide frequent feedback, call on the client often, arrange for a listening buddy).

12. Teach the client more effective test-taking strategies (e.g., study over an extended period of time, review material regularly, read directions twice, recheck work).

13. Instruct the parents on how to give proper directions (e.g., gain the client's attention, make one request at a time, clear away distractions, repeat instructions, and obtain frequent feedback from the client).

14. Teach the client mediational and self-control strategies (i.e., "stop, look, listen, and think") to delay

aggressive behaviors. (14, 16, 22, 27, 29)

18. Increase verbalizations by the client which he/she accepts responsibility for misbehavior. (14, 17, 19)

19. Decrease the frequency of arguments and physical fights with his/her siblings. (6, 14, 22, 23, 27)

20. Increase the frequency of positive self-statements. (24, 25)

21. Increase participation in extracurricular activities or positive peer group activities. (25, 26)

22. Increase positive interactions with peers. (24, 25, 26, 28)

23. Increase brain-wave control, which results in improved attention span and decreased impulsivity and hyperactivity. (29, 30)

___. _____
    _____

___. _____
    _____

___. _____
    _____

gratification and inhibit impulses.

15. Identify a variety of positive reinforcers or rewards to maintain the client's interest or motivation.

16. Conduct family therapy sessions to assist the parents in establishing clearly identified rules and boundaries.

17. Design a reward system and/or contract to reinforce the client's desired positive behaviors and deter impulsive behaviors.

18. Encourage the parents to utilize natural, logical consequences for the client's disruptive and negative attention-seeking behaviors.

19. Design a behavior modification program for the classroom to improve the client's academic performance, social skills, and impulse control.

20. Assign the client's parents to read *1-2-3 Magic: Training Your Preschoolers and Preteens to Do What You Want* (Phelan) or *Your Hyperactive Child* (Ingersoll); process the reading with the therapist.

21. Encourage the client's parents to participate in an ADHD support group.

22. Teach the client effective problem-solving skills (i.e., identify the problem, brainstorm alternate solutions,

select an option, implement a course of action, and evaluate).

23. Assign the client to read *Putting on the Brakes* (Quinn and Stern) or *Sometimes I Drive My Mom Crazy, But I Know She's Crazy About Me* (Shapiro); process the reading with the therapist.

24. Identify and reinforce positive behaviors to assist the client in establishing and maintaining friendships.

25. Encourage the client to participate in extracurricular or positive peer group activities to improve his/her social skills.

26. Arrange for the client to attend group therapy to build social skills.

27. Utilize the therapeutic game Stop, Relax & Think (Shapiro)* to assist the client in developing self-control.

28. Encourage the client to use self-monitoring checklists to improve attention, academic performance, and social skills.

29. Utilize brain-wave biofeedback techniques to improve the attention span, impulse control, and ability to relax.

---

* L. Shapiro, *Stop, Relax and Think* (King of Prussia, Pa.: Center for Applied Psychology, 1991).

30. Encourage the client to transfer the biofeedback training skills of relaxation and cognitive focusing to everyday situations (e.g., classroom and home).

___. _____

_____

___. _____

_____

___. _____

_____

DIAGNOSTIC SUGGESTIONS

Axis I:	314.01	Attention-Deficit/Hyperactivity Disorder, Combined Type
	314.00	Attention-Deficit/Hyperactivity Disorder, Predominantly Inattentive Type
	314.01	Attention-Deficit/Hyperactivity Disorder, Predominantly Hyperactive-Impulsive Type
	314.9	Attention-Deficit/Hyperactivity Disorder NOS
	312.81	Conduct Disorder/Childhood-Onset Type
	312.82	Conduct Disorder/Adolescent-Onset Type
	313.81	Oppositional Defiant Disorder
	312.9	Disruptive Behavior Disorder NOS
	296.xx	Bipolar I Disorder
	_____	_____
	_____	_____
Axis II:	V71.09	No Diagnosis
	799.9	Diagnosis Deferred
	_____	_____
	_____	_____

AUTISM/PERVASIVE DEVELOPMENTAL DISORDER

BEHAVIORAL DEFINITIONS

1. Pervasive lack of interest in or responsiveness to other people.
2. Chronic failure to develop social relationships appropriate to the developmental level.
3. Lack of spontaneity and emotional or social reciprocity.
4. Significant delays in or total lack of spoken language development and inability to sustain or initiate conversation.
5. Oddities in speech and language as manifested by echolalia, pronominal reversal, or metaphorical language.
6. Inflexible adherence to repetition of nonfunctional rituals or stereotyped motor mannerisms.
7. Persistent preoccupation with objects, parts of objects, or restricted areas of interest.
8. Marked impairment or extreme variability in intellectual and cognitive functioning.
9. Extreme resistance or overreaction to minor changes in routines or environment.
10. Emotional constriction or blunted affect.
11. Recurrent pattern of self-abusive behaviors (e.g., head banging, biting, or burning him/herself).

__. _____
   _____
__. _____
   _____

—. _____
_____

LONG-TERM GOALS

1. Achieve the educational, behavioral, and social goals identified on the client's Individualized Educational Plan (IEP).
2. Develop basic language skills and the ability to simply communicate with others.
3. Establish a basic bond between the client and primary attachment figures in his/her life.
4. Family members develop acceptance of the client's overall capabilities and place realistic expectations on his/her behavior.
5. Engage in reciprocal, cooperative, or imitative play on a regular basis.
6. Stabilize mood so that the client is able to tolerate changes in routine or environment.
7. Eliminate all self-abusive behaviors.

—. _____
_____

—. _____
_____

—. _____
_____

SHORT-TERM OBJECTIVES

1. Complete an intellectual and cognitive assessment. (1, 4)
2. Complete a speech/language evaluation. (2, 7, 10)
3. Complete a neurological evaluation and/or neuropsychological testing. (3, 4)
4. Take medication as prescribed by a psychiatrist. (3, 5)

THERAPEUTIC INTERVENTIONS

1. Arrange for an intellectual and cognitive assessment to gain greater insight into the client's learning strengths and weaknesses.
2. Refer the client for speech/language evaluation.
3. Arrange for neurological evaluation or neuropsychological testing of the client to rule out organic factors.

5. The client and his/her parents comply fully with the recommendations offered by the assessment(s) and Individualized Educational Planning Committee (IEPC). (1, 2, 6, 7, 22)

6. Comply with the move to an appropriate classroom setting. (1, 2, 6, 7)

7. Comply with the move to an appropriate alternative placement setting. (8, 15)

8. Increase the appropriate spontaneous verbalizations toward the therapist. (9, 11, 12, 13)

9. Decrease the oddities or peculiarities in speech and language. (10, 11, 12, 15)

10. Increase the frequency of communication or interaction with others. (9, 10, 11, 12, 13)

11. Decrease the frequency and severity of temper outbursts and erratic shifts in mood. (14, 15, 16)

12. Decrease the frequency and severity of self-abusive behaviors. (14, 17, 18)

13. Participate in play or work activity with the parents or sibling(s) for 20 minutes each day. (13, 19, 20, 21)

14. Develop basic or essential self-care and independent living skills. (25, 26, 28, 29)

15. The parents develop and maintain a positive support system. (22, 23, 24)

4. Provide feedback to the client's parents regarding all evaluation and assessment findings.

5. Arrange for psychiatric evaluation of the client.

6. Attend an IEPC meeting to determine the client's eligibility for special education services, design educational interventions, and establish goals.

7. Consult with the parents, teachers, and other appropriate school officials about designing effective learning programs or interventions that build on the client's strengths and compensate for weaknesses.

8. Consult with parents, school officials, and mental health professionals about the need to place the client in an alternative setting (e.g., foster care, group home, or residential program).

9. Actively build a level of trust with the client through consistent eye contact, frequent attention and interest, unconditional positive regard, and warm acceptance to facilitate increased communication.

10. Refer the client to a speech/language pathologist to improve his/her speech and language abilities.

11. Design and implement a response-shaping program

16. Develop basic job skills that allow the client to channel strengths or areas of interest in a positive manner. (27, 30)

—. _____
   _____
—. _____
   _____
—. _____
   _____

using positive reinforcement principles to facilitate the client's language development.

12. Provide the parents with encouragement, support, and methods to foster the client's language development.

13. Employ frequent use of praise and positive reinforcement to increase the client's acknowledgment and responsiveness to others' verbalizations.

14. Teach the parents behavioral management techniques (e.g., time-out, response cost, removal of privileges) to decrease the client's idiosyncratic speech, excessive self-stimulation, temper outbursts, and self-abusive behaviors.

15. Design a token economy for the classroom or residential program to improve the client's social skills, impulse control, and speech/language abilities.

16. Develop a reward system or contingency contract to improve the client's social skills and anger control.

17. Use aversive therapy techniques to stop or limit the client's self-abusive behaviors.

18. Counsel with the parents to develop interventions to manage the client's self-abusive behaviors using

positive reinforcement, response cost, and, if necessary, physical restraint.

19. Encourage family members to regularly include the client in structured work or play activities for 20 minutes each day.

20. Assign the client and his/her parents a task (e.g., swimming, riding a bike) that helps to build trust and mutual dependence.

21. Encourage detached parent(s) to increase their involvement in the client's daily life, leisure activities, or school work.

22. Educate the client's parents and family members about the symptoms and characteristics of autism or pervasive developmental disorder.

23. Encourage the client's parents to seek respite care on a periodic basis.

24. Refer the client's parents to a support group.

25. Counsel the parents about teaching the client essential self-care skills (e.g., combing hair, bathing, brushing teeth).

26. Monitor and provide frequent feedback on the client's progress toward developing self-care skills.

27. Refer the client to a sheltered workshop or vocational training program to develop basic job skills.

28. Refer the client to an independent living skills center.

29. Refer the client to a summer camp program to foster social contacts.

30. Redirect the client preoccupation with objects or a restricted area of interest in socially acceptable ways (e.g., the client learns to tune instruments or packs objects in a sheltered workshop).

___. _____

_____

___. _____

_____

___. _____

_____

DIAGNOSTIC SUGGESTIONS

Axis I:	299.00	Autistic Disorder
	299.80	Pervasive Developmental Disorder NOS
	299.80	Rett's Disorder
	299.10	Childhood Disintegrative Disorder
	299.80	Asperger's Disorder
	313.89	Reactive Attachment Disorder of Infancy or Early Childhood
	307.3	Stereotypic Movement Disorder
	295.xx	Schizophrenia
	_____	_____
	_____	_____
Axis II:	317	Mild Mental Retardation
	319	Mental Retardation, Severity Unspecified
	799.9	Diagnosis Deferred
	V71.09	No Diagnosis
	_____	_____
	_____	_____

CHEMICAL DEPENDENCE

BEHAVIORAL DEFINITIONS

1. Marked change in behavior, that is, withdrawal from family and close friends, a loss of interest in activities, low energy, sleeping more, or a drop in school grades.
2. Intoxication and/or drug use observed on two or more occasions.
3. Mood swings.
4. Absence from or tardiness at school on a regular basis.
5. Peer group change to one that is noticeably chemically oriented.
6. Poor self-image; self-description as a loser or failure; rarely makes eye contact when talking to others.
7. Predominantly negative or hostile outlook on life and other people.
8. Possession of drug paraphernalia.
9. Apprehension for stealing alcohol from a store, the home of friends, or parents.
10. Arrest for an MIP (Minor In Possession), OUIL/DUIL, or drunk and disorderly charge.
11. Positive family history of chemical dependence.
12. Self-report of daily use of a mood-altering substance or using until high on a regular basis.

___. _____
_____

___. _____
_____

___. _____
_____

LONG-TERM GOALS

1. Confirm or rule out the existence of chemical dependence.
2. Maintain total abstinence from all mood-altering substances while developing an active recovery program.
3. Reestablish sobriety while developing a plan for addressing relapse issues.
4. Confirm and address chemical dependence as a family issue.
5. Develop the skills essential to maintaining a life free from drugs and/or alcohol.
6. Reduce the level of family stress related to chemical dependence.
7. Reestablish connections with relationships and groups that will support and enhance ongoing recovery.
8. Develop an understanding of the pattern of relapse and strategies for coping effectively to help sustain long-term recovery.

—. _____
_____
—. _____
_____
—. _____
_____

SHORT-TERM OBJECTIVES

1. Complete an evaluation for chemical dependence. (1, 2, 6)

2. Acknowledge honestly (without denial) the pattern of chemical usage. (2, 3, 8, 12)

3. Comply with any requests for drug screens. (4, 6, 10, 11)

4. Complete a genogram that identifies members who are chemically dependent and family relationship patterns. (1, 2, 5)

THERAPEUTIC INTERVENTIONS

1. Arrange for a complete chemical dependence evaluation of the client.

2. Explore with the client the pattern of substance abuse.

3. Ask the client to discuss the pattern of substance abuse in group therapy sessions.

4. Arrange for and monitor all drug screens of the client.

5. Conduct family and individual sessions that develop a genogram.

5. Comply with all the recommendations of the chemical dependence evaluation. (1, 4, 6, 7)

6. Verbally acknowledge the pattern of addiction-related problems in the client's life. (3, 8, 9, 12)

7. Make a verbal agreement to attempt to terminate all mood-altering chemical use. (6, 10, 11)

8. Sign a written agreement to refrain from the use of alcohol until of the legal age. (4, 7, 10, 11)

9. Verbally acknowledge and accept the chemical dependence and the need for help. (3, 8, 9, 12)

10. Increase knowledge of the addiction and the process of recovery. (13, 14, 15, 19)

11. Verbally identify instances when an impulsive action led to negative consequences and describe how delay of the action may have been achieved. (14, 15, 18)

12. Develop key strategies for coping with family stressors and the dynamics that trigger use. (5, 18, 24, 27)

13. Verbalize the changes in lifestyle necessary to overcome chemical dependence. (21, 22, 25, 26)

14. Identify the family dynamics and stressors that are relapse triggers. (5, 14, 24, 25)

6. Present the recommendations of a chemical dependence evaluation to the client and his/her family and encourage compliance.

7. Assist the client and his/her family in finding appropriate treatment programs and support groups for recovery.

8. Assign the client to complete an Alcoholics Anonymous (AA) first-step paper and present it in group therapy or to therapist for feedback.

9. Ask the client to make a list of the ways chemical use has negatively impacted his/her life and process the list with the therapist or group.

10. Assist the client and his/her family in constructing and signing an agreement to refrain from using substances.

11. Develop an agreement with the client around terminating substance use; monitor the results and give feedback when appropriate.

12. Confront denial and assist the client in coming to an acceptance of his/her chemical dependence in individual or group sessions.

13. Assign the client to attend group therapy.

14. Assign the client to attend a chemical dependence didactic series to increase knowl-

15. Develop a list of personal relapse warning signs and strategies for coping effectively with each trigger. (27, 28, 29, 30)

16. Develop and commit to a written relapse contract with the family and/or significant others. (29, 30, 33, 34)

17. Identify the thoughts and feelings that lead to relapse. (24, 27, 28, 29)

18. Verbalize the details of the circumstances that led to the most recent relapse. (13, 29, 30, 32)

19. Develop a brief, personalized treatment plan for relapse prevention. (29, 30, 32, 33)

20. Each family member develop in writing his/her own relapse prevention plan for the client and share it with him/her. (35, 36, 40, 41)

21. Develop a written aftercare plan that supports maintaining sobriety. (14, 22, 25, 26)

22. Family members verbalize an understanding of their role in the disease and the process of recovery. (35, 36, 37, 40)

23. Family members decrease the frequency of enabling the chemically dependent child after verbally identifying their enabling behaviors. (35, 36, 37, 40)

edge of the patterns and effects of chemical dependence.

15. Require the client to attend all chemical dependence didactics, ask him/her to identify several key points attained from each didactic, and process these points with the therapist.

16. Assign the client to ask two or three people who are close to him/her to write a letter to the therapist in which they identify how they saw the client's chemical dependence negatively impacting his/her life; process these letters with the client.

17. Direct the client to write a good-bye letter to the drug of choice; read it and process the related feelings with the therapist.

18. Increase the client's awareness of impulsiveness by pointing out instances of such behavior and its consequences; assist in developing strategies for handling impulses.

19. Ask the client to read Ohm's pamphlet on marijuana or another specific cannabis-related article and process with the therapist five key points gained from the reading.

20. Require the client to read pages 1 to 52 in *Alcoholics Anonymous: The Big Book*

24. Family members develop the skills to implement the techniques involved in *tough love.* (35, 36, 38, 39)

__. _____
   _____
__. _____
   _____
__. _____
   _____

and gather five key points from it to process with the therapist.

21. Recommend that the client attend Narcotics Anonymous (NA) or Young People's AA meetings and report to the therapist the impact of the meetings.

22. Assign the client to meet with an NA or AA member who has been working with a 12-step program for several years and find out specifically how the program helped him/her stay sober; process the meeting with the client.

23. Encourage the client to find two temporary sponsors and meet with them weekly. The therapist should monitor and process the results.

24. Probe the client's feelings of depression and low self-esteem that may underlie chemical abuse.

25. Plan with the client how to develop drug-free peer group friendships that will support sobriety.

26. Encourage the client's involvement in extracurricular social, athletic, or artistic activities with a positive peer group that expands interests beyond hanging out.

27. Process feelings of rejection from the client's family and/or friends that could cause escape into chemical dependence.

28. Assist the client in developing strategies to cope effectively with family dynamics that trigger drug or alcohol use.

29. Direct the client to attend a group or lecture series on relapse.

30. Assist the client in identifying relapse signs and triggers and developing specific strategies for responding effectively to each.

31. Assign the client to read *It Will Never Happen to Me* (Black) and process five key items from the book with the therapist or group.

32. Help the client to become more skilled in recognizing, processing, and coping with thoughts and feelings.

33. Assign the client patient to write a personalized relapse prevention plan and process the plan with the therapist and sponsor.

34. Assign the client to write an aftercare plan and process it with the therapist and family.

35. Direct the client's family to attend Al-Anon, Nar-Anon, or Tough Love meetings.

36. Educate the client's family in the dynamics of enabling and tough love.

37. Ask the client's family to attend the family education component of the treatment program.

38. Monitor the client's family for enabling behaviors and redirect them in the family session as appropriate.

39. Assist the client's family members in implementing and sticking with tough love techniques.

40. Assign appropriate reading that will increase the family members' knowledge of the disease and recovery process, e.g., *Bradshaw on the Family* (Bradshaw), *Adult Children of Alcoholics* (Woititz), *It Will Never Happen to Me* (Black).

41. Help the family members develop their own individual relapse prevention plans for the client and facilitate a session where plans are shared with the chemically dependent member.

__. _____

_____

__. _____

_____

__. _____

_____

DIAGNOSTIC SUGGESTIONS

Axis I:

305.00	Alcohol Abuse
303.90	Alcohol Dependence
305.20	Cannabis Abuse
304.30	Cannabis Dependence
304.20	Cocaine Dependence
304.50	Hallucinogen Dependence
305.30	Hallucinogen Abuse
304.60	Inhalant Dependence
305.90	Inhalant Abuse
313.81	Oppositional Defiant Disorder
312.81	Conduct Disorder/Childhood-Onset Type
312.82	Conduct Disorder/Adolescent-Onset Type
300.4	Dysthymic Disorder
309.4	Adjustment Disorder With Mixed Disturbance of Emotions and Conduct
_____	_____
_____	_____

Axis II:

799.9	Diagnosis Deferred
V71.09	No Diagnosis
_____	_____
_____	_____

CONDUCT DISORDER/DELINQUENCY

BEHAVIORAL DEFINITIONS

1. Persistent failure to comply with rules or expectations in the home, school, or community.
2. Excessive fighting, intimidation of others, cruelty or violence toward people or animals, and destruction of property.
3. History of breaking and entering or stealing.
4. School adjustment characterized by repeated truancy, disrespectful attitude, and suspensions for misbehavior.
5. Repeated conflict or confrontations with authority figures at home, school, or in the community.
6. Failure to consider the consequences of actions, taking inappropriate risks, and engaging in thrill-seeking behaviors.
7. Numerous attempts to deceive others through lying, conning, or manipulating.
8. Consistent failure to accept responsibility for misbehavior, accompanied by a pattern of blaming others.
9. Little or no remorse for past misbehavior.
10. Lack of sensitivity to the thoughts, feelings, and needs of other people.
11. Multiple sexual partners, lack of emotional commitment, and engaging in sexual relations that increase the risk for contracting sexually transmitted diseases.

—. _____
_____

—. _____
_____

—. _____
_____

LONG-TERM GOALS

1. Demonstrate increased honesty, compliance with rules, sensitivity to the feelings and rights of others, control over impulses, and acceptance of responsibility for his/her behavior.
2. Comply with rules and expectations in the home, school, and community on a consistent basis.
3. Eliminate all illegal and antisocial behaviors.
4. Terminate all acts of violence or cruelty toward people or animals and the destruction of property.
5. Express anger through appropriate verbalizations and healthy physical outlets on a consistent basis.
6. Demonstrate marked improvement in impulse control.
7. Resolve the core conflicts which contribute to the emergence of conduct problems.
8. The parents establish and maintain appropriate parent-child boundaries, setting firm, consistent limits when the client acts out in an aggressive or rebellious manner.
9. Demonstrate empathy, concern, and sensitivity for the thoughts, feelings, and needs of others on a regular basis.
10. Eliminate all sexually promiscuous behaviors.

—. _____
   _____
—. _____
   _____
—. _____
   _____

SHORT-TERM OBJECTIVES

1. Complete psychological testing. (1, 3)
2. Complete a psychoeducational evaluation. (2, 3)
3. Complete a substance abuse evaluation and comply with the recommendations offered by the evaluation findings. (4, 5, 6)

THERAPEUTIC INTERVENTIONS

1. Arrange for psychological testing of the client to assess whether emotional factors or ADHD are contributing to his/her impulsivity and acting-out behaviors.
2. Arrange for a psychoeducational evaluation of the

4. Cooperate with the recommendations or requirements mandated by the criminal justice system. (3, 5, 6, 7)

5. Move to an appropriate alternative setting or juvenile detention facility. (5, 6, 7)

6. Recognize and verbalize how feelings are connected to misbehavior. (9, 11, 35)

7. Increase the number of statements that reflect the acceptance of responsibility for misbehavior. (10, 22, 12, 13)

8. Decrease the frequency of verbalizations that project the blame for the problems onto other people. (10, 12, 13)

9. Express anger through appropriate verbalization and healthy physical outlets. (14, 15, 16, 17)

10. Reduce the frequency and severity of aggressive, destructive, and antisocial behaviors. (8, 10, 14, 16)

11. Increase the compliance with rules at home and school. (8, 9, 19, 20, 21)

12. Postpone recreational activity (e.g., playing basketball with friends) until after completing homework or chores. (8, 18, 22, 23)

13. The parents establish appropriate boundaries, develop clear rules, and fol-

client to rule out the presence of a learning disability that may be contributing to the impulsivity and acting-out behaviors in the school setting.

3. Provide feedback to the client, his/her parents, school officials, or criminal justice officials regarding psychological and/or psychoeducational testing.

4. Arrange for substance abuse evaluation and/or treatment for the client.

5. Consult with criminal justice officials about the appropriate consequences for the client's antisocial behaviors (e.g., pay restitution, community service, probation, intensive surveillance).

6. Consult with the parents, school officials, and criminal justice officials about the need to place the client in an alternative setting (e.g., foster home, group home, residential program, or juvenile detention facility).

7. Encourage and challenge the parents not to protect the client from the legal consequences of his/her antisocial behaviors.

8. Assist the client's parents in establishing clearly defined rules, boundaries, and consequences for misbehavior.

low through consistently with consequences for mis-behavior. (8, 20, 21, 23)

14. The client and his/her parents agree to and follow through with the implementation of a reward system or contingency contract. (8, 20, 22)

15. The parents increase the frequency of praise and positive reinforcement to the client. (20, 22)

16. Increase the time spent with the uninvolved or detached parent(s) in leisure, school, or work activities. (24, 25, 26, 27)

17. The parents verbalize appropriate boundaries for discipline to prevent further occurrences of abuse and ensure the safety of the client and his/her siblings. (25, 28, 29, 30)

18. Verbalize an understanding of how current acting-out and aggressive behaviors are associated with past neglect, abuse, separation, or abandonment. (28, 31, 32, 33, 34)

19. Identify and verbally express feelings associated with past neglect, abuse, separation, or abandonment. (31, 32, 33, 34, 35)

20. Increase participation in extracurricular activities or positive peer group activities. (36, 38, 39)

9. Actively build the level of trust with the client in therapy sessions through consistent eye contact, active listening, unconditional positive regard, and warm acceptance to help increase his/her ability to identify and express feelings.

10. Firmly confront the client's antisocial behavior and attitude, pointing out consequences for him/herself and others.

11. Assist the client in making a connection between feelings and reactive behaviors.

12. Confront statements in which the client blames others for his/her misbehavior and fails to accept responsibility for his/her actions.

13. Explore and process the factors that contribute to the client's pattern of blaming others.

14. Teach mediational and self-control strategies (e.g., relaxation, "stop, look, listen, and think") to help the client express anger through appropriate verbalizations and healthy physical outlets.

15. Encourage the client to use self-monitoring checklists at home or school to develop more effective anger and impulse control.

21. Identify and verbalize how acting-out behaviors negatively affect others. (10, 13, 37)

22. Increase verbalizations of empathy and concern for other people. (18, 35, 36, 37)

23. Establish and maintain steady employment to deter impulsive behaviors. (40, 41)

24. Identify and verbalize the risks involved in sexually promiscuous behaviors. (42, 43)

25. Identify and verbalize the feelings, irrational beliefs, and needs that contribute to sexually promiscuous behaviors. (28, 42, 43)

26. Increase communication, intimacy, and consistency between the parents. (24, 25, 44)

27. Take medication as prescribed by the physician. (1, 45)

__. _____
    _____

__. _____
    _____

__. _____
    _____

16. Utilize the therapeutic workbook, *The Angry Monster* (Shore), to help the client develop more effective anger and impulse control.

17. Teach the client effective communication and assertiveness skills to express feelings in a controlled fashion and meet his/her needs through more constructive actions.

18. Assist the parents in increasing structure to help the client learn to delay gratification for longer-term goals (e.g., complete homework or chores before playing basketball).

19. Establish clear rules for the client in home or school; ask him/her to repeat the rules to demonstrate an understanding of the expectations.

20. Design a reward system and/or contingency contract for the client to reinforce identified positive behaviors and deter impulsive behaviors.

21. Design and implement a token economy to increase the client's positive social behaviors and deter impulsive, acting-out behaviors.

22. Encourage the parents to provide frequent praise and positive reinforcement for the client's positive social behaviors and good impulse control.

23. Assign the client's parents to read *1-2-3 Magic: Training Your Preschooler and Preteens to Do What You Want* (Phelan), *Family Rules* (Kaye), and *Assertive Discipline for Parents* (Canter and Canter).

24. Conduct family therapy sessions to explore the dynamics that contribute to the emergence of the client's behavioral problems.

25. Utilize the family-sculpting technique in which the client defines the roles and behaviors of each family member in a scene of his/her choosing to assess the family dynamics.

26. Conduct a family therapy session in which the client's family members are given a task or problem to solve together (e.g., build a craft); observe family interactions and process the experience with them afterward.

27. Give a directive to uninvolved or disengaged parent(s) to spend more time with the client in leisure, school, or work activities.

28. Explore the client's family background for a history of physical, sexual, or substance abuse, which may contribute to his/her behavioral problems.

29. Confront the client's parents to cease physically abusive or overly punitive methods of discipline.

30. Implement the steps necessary to protect the client or siblings from further abuse (e.g., report abuse to the appropriate agencies; remove the client or perpetrator from the home).

31. Encourage and support the client in expressing feelings associated with neglect, abuse, separation, or abandonment.

32. Conduct individual play therapy sessions to provide the client with the opportunity to express feelings surrounding past neglect, abuse, separation, or abandonment.

33. Interpret the feelings expressed in play therapy and relate them to the client's anger and acting-out behaviors.

34. Assign the client the task of writing a letter to an absent parent or use the empty-chair technique to assist the client in expressing and working through feelings of anger and sadness about past abandonment.

35. Utilize the therapeutic game, Talking, Feeling, Doing,* to increase the client's awareness of his/her thoughts and feelings.

---

* Creative Therapeutics, Cresskill, New Jersey, 1973.

36. Arrange for the client to participate in group therapy to improve his/her social judgment and interpersonal skills.

37. Assign the client the task of showing empathy, kindness, or sensitivity to the needs of others (e.g., read a bedtime story to a sibling, mow the lawn for the grandmother).

38. Encourage the client to participate in extracurricular or positive peer group activities to provide a healthy outlet for anger, improve social skills, and increase self-esteem.

39. Refer the client to the Big Brothers/Big Sisters organization to provide a positive role model.

40. Refer the client to vocational training to develop basic job skills and find employment.

41. Encourage and reinforce the client's acceptance of the responsibility of a job, the authority of a supervisor, and the employer's rules.

42. Provide the client with sex education and discuss the risks involved with sexually promiscuous behaviors.

43. Explore the client's feelings, irrational beliefs, and unmet needs that contribute to the emergence of sexually promiscuous behaviors.

44. Assess the marital dyad for possible conflict and triangulation that places the focus on the client's acting-out behaviors and away from marriage issues.

45. Arrange for a medication evaluation of the client to improve his/her impulse control and stabilize moods.

___. _____

_____

___. _____

_____

___. _____

_____

DIAGNOSTIC SUGGESTIONS

Axis I:

312.81	Conduct Disorder/Childhood-Onset Type
312.82	Conduct Disorder/Adolescent-Onset Type
313.81	Oppositional Defiant Disorder
312.9	Disruptive Behavioral Disorder NOS
314.01	Attention-Deficit/Hyperactive Disorder, Predominantly Hyperactive-Impulsive Type
314.9	Attention-Deficit/Hyperactivity Disorder NOS
312.34	Intermittent Explosive Disorder
V71.02	Child or Adolescent Antisocial Behavior
V61.20	Parent-Child Relational Problem
_____	_____
_____	_____

Axis II:

V71.09	No Diagnosis on Axis II
799.9	Diagnosis Deferred
_____	_____
_____	_____

DEPRESSION

BEHAVIORAL DEFINITIONS

1. Sad or flat affect.
2. Preoccupation with the subject of death.
3. Suicidal thoughts and/or actions.
4. Moody irritability.
5. Isolation from family and/or peers.
6. Deterioration of academic performance.
7. Lack of interest in previously enjoyed activities.
8. Refusal to communicate openly.
9. Use of street drugs to elevate mood.
10. Low energy.
11. Little or no eye contact and frequent verbalizations of low self-esteem.
12. Reduced appetite.
13. Increased sleep.
14. Poor concentration and indecision.
15. Feelings of hopelessness, worthlessness, or inappropriate guilt.
16. Unresolved grief issues.
17. Mood-related hallucinations or delusions.

___. _____
_____

___. _____
_____

___. _____
_____

LONG-TERM GOALS

1. Acknowledge the depression verbally and resolve its causes, leading to normalization of the emotional state.
2. Elevate the mood and show evidence of the usual energy, activities, and socialization level.
3. Reduce irritability and increase normal social interaction with family and friends.
4. Show a renewed typical interest in academic achievement, social involvement, and eating patterns as well as occasional expressions of joy and zest for life.

—. _____

_____

—. _____

_____

—. _____

_____

SHORT-TERM OBJECTIVES

1. Complete psychological testing to evaluate the depth of the depression. (1, 2)
2. State the connection between rebellion, self-destruction, or withdrawal and the underlying depression. (3, 4)
3. Verbally acknowledge unhappiness with life. (5, 7, 14, 15, 29)
4. Specify what is missing from life to cause the unhappiness. (5, 6, 8, 14, 15)
5. Specify what in the past or present life contributes to sadness. (5, 9, 10, 14, 15)

THERAPEUTIC INTERVENTIONS

1. Arrange for the administration of psychological testing to facilitate a more complete assessment of the depth of the client's depression.
2. Give feedback to the client (and his/her family) regarding psychological testing results.
3. Assess the client's level of self-understanding about self-defeating behaviors linked to the depression.
4. Interpret the client's acting-out behaviors as a reflection of the depression.

6. Assertively state to the therapist what is needed to be truly happy. (5, 10, 13, 29)

7. Express emotional needs to the significant others. (6, 11, 12, 28)

8. Stop the verbalized interest in the subject of death. (6, 7, 14, 15, 18)

9. Terminate suicidal behaviors and/or verbalizations of the desire to die. (16, 17, 18, 19)

10. Initiate and respond actively to social communication with the family and peers. (12, 20, 21, 28, 29)

11. Verbalize a feeling of being loved and accepted by family and friends. (6, 16, 17)

12. Describe an interest and participation in social and recreational activities. (13, 20)

13. Reduce anger and irritability as evidenced by friendly, pleasant interaction with family and friends. (11, 12, 20)

14. Cooperate with an evaluation of the necessity for psychotropic medications. (21, 22)

15. Take prescribed medications as directed by the physician. (21, 22, 23)

16. Improve academic performance evidenced by better grades and positive teacher reports. (24, 25)

5. Reinforce the client's open expression of underlying feelings of anger, hurt, and disappointment.

6. Probe the client's fears regarding the loss of love from others.

7. Confront the client's acting-out behaviors as avoidance of the real conflict with unmet emotional needs.

8. Ask the client to discuss what is missing from his/her life that contributes to the unhappiness.

9. Probe present aspects of the client's life that contribute to the sadness.

10. Explore the emotional pain from the client's past that contributes to the feelings of hopelessness and low self-esteem.

11. Hold a family therapy session to facilitate the expression of conflict with family members.

12. Support the client's expression of emotional needs to family members and significant others.

13. Urge the client to formulate a plan that leads to taking action to meet his/her needs.

14. Arrange for a play-therapy setting that allows the client to express feelings toward him/herself and others.

17. Eat nutritional meals regularly without strong urging from others. (21, 22, 23, 26)

18. Adjust sleep hours to those typical of the developmental stage. (21, 22, 23, 27)

__. _____
_____

__. _____
_____

__. _____
_____

15. Interpret the feelings expressed in play therapy as those of the client toward real life.

16. Assess the cognitive messages that the client gives to him/herself that reinforce helplessness and hopelessness.

17. Teach and reinforce positive cognitive messages that facilitate the growth of the client's self-confidence and self-acceptance.

18. Monitor the potential for self-harm and refer the client to a protective setting if necessary.

19. Contract with the client for no self-harm.

20. Encourage the client's participation in social/recreational activities that enrich life.

21. Assess the client's need for psychotropic medications.

22. Arrange for a prescription of antidepressant medications for the client.

23. Monitor medication effectiveness and side effects.

24. Challenge and encourage the client's academic effort.

25. Arrange for a tutor to increase the client's sense of academic mastery.

26. Monitor and encourage the client's food consumption.

27. Monitor the client's sleep patterns and the restfulness of sleep.

28. Work with the parents to develop their abilities to encourage, support, and tolerate the client's expression of his/her thoughts and feelings.

29. Use one of the therapeutic feelings games (e.g., Talking, Feeling, Doing)* to assist the client in being more verbal.

___. _____

_____

___. _____

_____

___. _____

_____

DIAGNOSTIC SUGGESTIONS

Axis I:	300.4	Dysthymic Disorder
	296.2x	Major Depressive Disorder, Single Episode
	296.3x	Major Depressive Disorder, Recurrent
	296.89	Bipolar II Disorder
	296.xx	Bipolar I Disorder
	301.13	Cyclothymic Disorder
	309.0	Adjustment Disorder With Depressed Mood
	310.1	Personality Change Due to (Axis III Disorder)
	V62.82	Bereavement
	_____	_____
	_____	_____
Axis II:	799.9	Diagnosis Deferred
	V71.09	No Diagnosis
	_____	_____
	_____	_____

---

* Creative Therapeutics, Cresskill, New Jersey, 1973.

EATING DISORDER

BEHAVIORAL DEFINITIONS

1. Rapid consumption of large quantities of food in a short time followed by self-induced vomiting and/or the use of laxatives due to the fear of weight gain.
2. Extreme weight loss (and amenorrhea in females) with a refusal to maintain a minimal healthy weight due to very limited ingestion of food and high frequency of secretive self-induced vomiting, inappropriate use of laxatives, and/or excessive strenuous exercise.
3. Preoccupation with body image related to a grossly unrealistic assessment of the self as being too fat or a strong denial of seeing the self as emaciated.
4. Irrational fear of becoming overweight.
5. Fluid and electrolyte imbalance.
6. Threat to life due to inadequate nutrition, fluid and electrolyte imbalance, and a general weakening of body systems resulting from self-induced vomiting, use of laxatives, and/or avoidance of eating enough nutritional food.

—. _____
_____

—. _____
_____

—. _____
_____

LONG-TERM GOALS

1. Restore normal eating patterns, body weight, balanced fluid and electrolytes, and a realistic perception of body size.

2. Terminate the pattern of binge eating and purging behavior with a return to normal eating of enough nutritious foods to maintain a healthy weight.

3. Stabilize the medical condition, resume patterns of food intake that will sustain life, and gain weight to a normal level.

4. Gain sufficient insight into the cognitive and emotional struggle to allow termination of the eating disorder and responsible maintenance of nutritional food intake.

5. Develop alternate coping strategies (i.e., feeling identification, assertiveness) to deal with underlying emotional issues, making the eating disorder unnecessary.

6. Gain awareness of the interconnectedness of low self-esteem and societal pressures with dieting, binge eating, and purging, in order to eliminate eating-disorder behaviors.

7. Change the definition of the self, so that it does not focus on weight, size, and shape as the primary criteria for self-acceptance.

8. Restructure the distorted thoughts, beliefs, and values that contribute to eating-disorder development.

—. _____

_____

—. _____

_____

—. _____

_____

SHORT-TERM OBJECTIVES

THERAPEUTIC INTERVENTIONS

1. Cooperate with a full physical and dental exam. (1, 2)

2. Cooperate with admission to inpatient treatment if a fragile medical condition necessitates such treatment. (1, 3)

3. Attain and maintain balanced fluids and electrolytes as well as resuming reproductive functions. (3, 4, 5, 9)

1. Refer the client to a physician for a thorough physical exam.

2. Refer the client to a dentist for a dental exam.

3. Refer the client for hospitalization, as necessary, if his/her weight loss becomes severe and physical health is jeopardized.

4. Establish a minimum daily caloric intake for the client.

4. Eat at regular intervals (three meals a day), consuming at least the minimum daily calories necessary to progressively gain weight. (4, 5, 6, 7, 8, 35)

5. Terminate inappropriate laxative use. (6, 9, 10, 11)

6. Terminate self-induced vomiting or alternate means of purging. (7, 8, 9, 10, 12)

7. Keep a daily journal of activities, thoughts, and feelings, noting any association with eating behavior. (7, 8, 12, 13)

8. Identify irrational beliefs about eating normal amounts of food. (11, 13, 14, 16, 37)

9. Verbalize the acceptance of full responsibility for choices about eating behavior. (9, 11, 29, 30, 36)

10. Stop hoarding food. (9, 10, 12, 29, 30)

11. Set reasonable limits on physical exercise. (7, 9, 11, 12)

12. Accept the responsibility for nutrition as shown by progressive weight gain or maintenance of an adequate weight without supervision. (10, 11, 17, 35, 36)

13. Identify irrational beliefs and expectations regarding body size. (12, 13, 14)

5. Assist the client in meal planning.

6. Monitor the client's weight and give realistic feedback regarding body thinness.

7. Assign the client to keep a journal of food intake, thoughts, and feelings.

8. Process the journal information with the therapist.

9. Monitor the client's vomiting frequency, food hoarding, exercise levels, and laxative usage.

10. Reinforce the client's weight gain and acceptance of personal responsibility for normal food intake.

11. Refer the client to a support group for eating disorders.

12. Assist in the identification of negative cognitive messages (e.g., catastrophizing, exaggerating) that mediate the client's avoidance of food intake.

13. Train the client to establish realistic cognitive messages regarding food intake and body size.

14. Confront the client's unrealistic assessment of his/her body image and assign exercises (e.g., positive self-talk in the mirror, shopping for clothes that flatter the appearance) that reinforce a healthy, realistic body appraisal.

15. Confront the client's irrational perfectionism in body image expectations and

14. Verbalize a realistic appraisal of weight status and body size. (12, 13, 14, 15, 35)

15. Verbalize the feelings of low self-esteem, depression, loneliness, anger, need for nurturance, or lack of trust that underlie the eating disorder. (7, 8, 11, 16, 19)

16. Acknowledge and overcome the role that passive-aggressive control (e.g., the refusal to accept guidance) has in the avoidance of eating. (16, 17, 18)

17. Disclose to family members the feelings of ambivalence regarding control and dependency and state how these feelings have affected eating patterns. (17, 18, 19)

18. Verbalize how the fear of sexual identity and development has influenced severe weight loss. (20, 21)

19. Verbalize the acceptance of sexual impulses and a desire for intimacy. (20, 21)

20. Identify the relationship between the fear of failure, the drive for perfectionism, and the roots of low self-esteem. (22, 23)

21. Verbalize the acceptance of shortcomings and normal failures as part of the human condition. (22, 23)

22. Acknowledge and resolve separation anxiety related to the emancipation process. (24, 25)

assist in his/her reasonable acceptance of the body with flaws.

16. Probe the client's emotional struggles that are camouflaged by the eating disorder.

17. Process the issue of passive-aggressive control in the client's rebellion against authority figures.

18. Discuss the issues of control of food as related to the client's fear of losing control of eating or weight.

19. Facilitate family therapy sessions that focus on owning feelings, clarifying messages, identifying control conflicts, and developing age-appropriate boundaries.

20. Process the client's fears regarding sexual development and sexual impulses.

21. Discuss the client's fear of losing control of sexual impulses and how the fear relates to keeping him/herself unattractively thin or fat.

22. Discuss the client's fear of failure and the role of perfectionism in the search for control and the avoidance of failure.

23. Reinforce the client's positive qualities and successes to reduce the fear of failure and build a positive sense of self.

24. Discuss the client's fear of independence and emancipation from parent figures.

23. Acknowledge to family members the feelings of fear related to separation and state the need for them to begin the letting-go process. (24, 25)

24. Develop assertive behaviors that allow for the healthy expression of needs and emotions. (26, 27)

25. State a basis for positive identity that is not based on weight and appearance but on character, traits, relationships, and intrinsic value. (23, 32, 33)

26. Verbalize the connection between suppressed emotional expression, difficulty with interpersonal issues, and unhealthy food usage. (26, 27)

27. Replace the food used for bingeing that was to be shared with others. (28, 29, 30)

28. Clean up after bingeing and purging episodes. (28, 29)

29. Parents state a detachment from responsibility for the client's eating disorder. (30, 31)

30. Understand and verbalize the connection between too-restrictive dieting and binge episodes. (34, 35, 36, 37)

—. _____

_____

25. Hold family therapy sessions that focus on issues of separation, dependency, and emancipation.

26. Train the client in assertiveness or refer him/her to an assertiveness training class.

27. Reinforce the client's assertiveness behaviors in the session and reports of successful assertiveness between sessions.

28. Confront the client regarding the impact of bingeing and purging behavior on household members and the need for consideration of their feelings and rights.

29. Assist the parents in developing a behavioral contract with the client in which the client pays a consequence (e.g., added household chores or loss of money, privilege, or curfew time) for bingeing on family food, hoarding food, or failing to clean up after purging.

30. Teach parents how to successfully detach from taking responsibility for the client's eating behavior without becoming hostile or indifferent.

31. Recommend that the client's parents or friends read *Surviving an Eating Disorder* (Siegel, et al.) and process the concepts in a family therapy session.

___. _____
      _____
___. _____
      _____

32. Assist the client in identifying a basis for self-worth apart from body image by reviewing his/her talents, successes, positive traits, importance to others, and intrinsic spiritual value.

33. Assign the client the book *Body Traps* (Rodin) and process the key ideas regarding obsessing over body image.

34. Assist the client in understanding the relationship between bingeing and lack of regular mealtimes or total deprivation from specific foods.

35. Establish healthy weight goals for the client per the Body Mass Index (BMI = pounds of body weight × 700/height in inches/height in inches; normal range is 20 to 27 and below 18 is medically critical),* the Metropolitan Height and Weight Tables†, or some other recognized standard.

36. Refer the client to a dietitian for education in healthy eating and nutritional concerns.

37. Encourage the client to read book(s) on binge eating (e.g., *Overcoming Binge Eating* by Fairburn) to

---

* G. T. Wilson, C. G. Fairburn, and W. S. Agras, "Cognitive-Behavioral Therapy for Bulimia Nervosa" in D. M. Garner and P. Garfinkel (eds.), *Handbook of Treatment for Eating Disorders* (New York: Guilford Press, 199—).
† Metropolitan Height and Weight Tables (New York: Metropolitan Life Insurance Company, Health and Safety Division, 1983).

increase the awareness of
the components of eating
disorders.

—. _____

_____

—. _____

_____

—. _____

_____

DIAGNOSTIC SUGGESTIONS

Axis I: 307.1   Anorexia Nervosa
              307.51   Bulimia Nervosa
              307.50   Eating Disorder NOS
              300.4   Dysthymic Disorder

              _____   _____

              _____   _____

Axis II: 799.9   Diagnosis Deferred
              V71.09   No Diagnosis
              301.6   Dependent Personality Disorder

              _____   _____

              _____   _____

ENURESIS/ENCOPRESIS

BEHAVIORAL DEFINITIONS

1. Repeated pattern of voluntary or involuntary voiding of urine into bed or clothes during the day or at night, after an age of five when continence is expected.
2. Repeated passage of feces, whether voluntary or involuntary, into inappropriate places (e.g., clothing or floor) after an age of five when continence is expected.
3. Feelings of shame associated with enuresis or encopresis that cause the avoidance of situations (e.g., overnight visits with friends) that might lead to further embarrassment.
4. Social ridicule, isolation, or ostracism by peers because of enuresis or encopresis.
5. Frequent attempts to hide feces or soiled clothing because of shame or fear of further ridicule, criticism, or punishment.
6. Excessive anger, rejection, or punishment by the parent(s) or caretaker(s) centering around toilet-training practices, which contributes to low self-esteem.
7. Strong feelings of fear or hostility, which are channeled into acts of enuresis and encopresis.
8. Deliberate smearing of feces in inappropriate places.

—. _____

_____

—. _____

_____

—. _____

_____

LONG-TERM GOALS

1. Eliminate all diurnal and/or nocturnal episodes of enuresis.
2. Terminate all episodes of encopresis, whether voluntary or involuntary.
3. Resolve the underlying core conflicts contributing to the emergence of enuresis or encopresis.
4. Eliminate rigid and coercive toilet-training practices by the parents.
5. Eradicate the hostile-dependent cycle in the family system, in which the soiling or wetting angers the parents, the parents respond in an overly critical or hostile manner, and then the client "punishes" the parents for their anger by soiling or wetting.

__. _____

_____

__. _____

_____

__. _____

_____

SHORT-TERM OBJECTIVES

1. Comply with the physician's orders for medical tests and medications. (1, 2, 3)
2. Take prescribed medication as directed by the physician. (2, 3)
3. Complete psychological testing. (4, 23, 24)
4. Parents consistently comply with the use of bell-and-pad conditioning procedures to treat nocturnal enuresis. (5, 6, 8, 9)
5. Reduce the frequency of enuretic behavior. (5, 6, 7, 8, 9)

THERAPEUTIC INTERVENTIONS

1. Refer the client for a medical examination to rule out organic or physical causes of the enuresis or encopresis.
2. Arrange for a medication evaluation of the client.
3. Monitor the client for compliance, side effects, and overall effectiveness of the medications. Consult with the prescribing physician at regular intervals.
4. Arrange for psychological testing to rule out the presence of serious, underlying emotional problems; pro-

6. Reduce the frequency of encopretic behavior. (6, 10)

7. Increase the client's role in implementing toilet-training practices and interventions. (11, 12, 15)

8. Identify the negative social consequences that may occur from peers if enuresis or encopresis continues. (11, 12, 15)

9. Verbalize how anxiety or fears associated with toilet-training practices are unrealistic or irrational. (13, 14)

10. Overly critical parent(s) verbally recognize how rigid toilet-training practices or hostile, critical remarks contribute to the client's enuresis or encopresis. (16, 17, 18, 19)

11. Decrease the frequency and severity of hostile, critical remarks by the parents regarding the client's toilet training. (16, 18, 19, 22)

12. Increase the parent(s)' empathic responses to the client's thoughts, feelings, and needs. (17, 19, 21, 31)

13. Increase the disengaged parent's involvement in toilet-training practices. (17, 20)

14. Strengthen the relationship with the disengaged parent as demonstrated by increased time spent between the client and parent. (17, 21)

vide feedback on the testing to the client and his/her parents.

5. Train the client and his/her parents to treat enuresis by using bell-and-pad conditioning procedures in which a urine-sensitive pad causes an alarm to sound when involuntary wetting occurs.

6. Design and counsel the parents on the use of positive reinforcement procedures to increase the client's bladder or bowel control.

7. Teach the client and his/her parents effective bladder retention training techniques that increase the client's awareness of the sensation or need to urinate.

8. Train the client's parents or caretakers on the use of staggered-awakening procedures, utilizing a variable-interval schedule, to control nocturnal enuresis.

9. Design and implement dry-bed techniques, training the parents and the client in response inhibition, positive reinforcement, rapid awakening, increasing fluid intake, self-correction of accidents, and decreased critical comments about toilet-training behavior.

10. Train the client and his/her parents how to implement a systematic operant-

15. Understand and verbally recognize the secondary gain that results from enuresis or encopresis. (22, 23, 31)

16. Verbalize how enuresis or encopresis is associated with past separation, loss, trauma, or rejection experiences. (24, 25, 26)

17. Identify and express feelings associated with past separation, loss, trauma, or rejection experiences. (24, 25, 26, 27)

18. Decrease the frequency of self-descriptive statements that reflect feelings of low self-esteem, shame, or embarrassment. (29, 30)

19. Increase the frequency of positive self-descriptive statements that reflect improved self-esteem. (29, 30)

20. Appropriately express anger verbally and physically rather than channeling anger through enuresis or encopresis. (27, 28)

___. _____

_____

___. _____

_____

___. _____

_____

conditioning program, which combines positive reinforcement techniques with the use of glycerine suppositories and enemas if the client does not defecate voluntarily each day.

11. Encourage and challenge the client to assume active responsibility in achieving mastery of bladder and/or bowel control (i.e., keep a record of wet and dry days, set an alarm clock for voiding times, clean soiled underwear or linens).

12. Challenge and/or confront the client's lack of motivation or compliance in following through with recommended therapeutic interventions.

13. Explore irrational cognitive messages that produce fear or anxiety in the client associated with toilet training.

14. Assist the client in realizing how anxiety or fears associated with toilet training are irrational or unrealistic.

15. Identify and discuss negative social consequences the client may experience from peers, in order to increase his/her motivation to master bladder/bowel control.

16. Counsel the client's parents on effective toilet-training practices.

17. Conduct family therapy sessions to assess the dynamics that contribute to the emergence or reinforcement of the client's enuresis or encopresis.

18. Explore parent-child interactions to assess whether the parents' toilet-training practices are excessively rigid or if the parents make frequent, hostile, critical remarks about the client.

19. Confront and challenge the parent(s) about making overly critical or hostile remarks that contribute to the client's low self-esteem, shame and embarrassment, and anger.

20. Assign the disengaged parent the responsibility of overseeing or teaching the client effective toilet-training practices (e.g., keep a record of wet and dry days, gently awaken the client for bladder voiding, remind or teach the client how to clean soiled underwear or linens).

21. Give a directive to the disengaged parent to spend quality time with the client (e.g., work on homework together, go to the park, or engage in a sporting activity).

22. Assess parent-child interactions for the presence of a hostile-dependent cycle where the client's wetting

or soiling angers the parents, the parents respond in an overly critical or hostile manner, the client seeks to "punish" the parents for their strong display of anger, and so on.

23. Assist the client and his/her parents in developing insight into the secondary gain received from enuresis or encopresis.

24. Assess whether the client's enuresis or encopresis is associated with past separation, loss, traumatization, or rejection experiences.

25. Explore, encourage, and support the client in verbally expressing and clarifying feelings associated with past separation, loss, trauma, or rejection experiences.

26. Utilize individual play therapy sessions to provide the client with the opportunity to express and work through feelings associated with past separation, loss, trauma, or rejection experiences.

27. Teach the client effective communication and assertiveness skills to improve his/her ability to express thoughts and feelings through appropriate verbalizations.

28. Teach the client appropriate physical outlets, which allow the expression of

anger in a constructive manner rather than channeling anger through inappropriate wetting or soiling.

29. Identify and list the client's positive characteristics to help decrease feelings of shame and embarrassment; reinforce the client's positive self-statements.

30. Assign the client to make one positive self-statement daily and record that in a journal.

31. Use a strategic family therapy approach, in which the therapist does not talk about enuresis or encopresis but discusses what might surface if this problem were resolved (i.e., camouflaged problems may be revealed).

—. _____
_____

—. _____
_____

—. _____
_____

DIAGNOSTIC SUGGESTIONS

Axis I:	307.6	Enuresis (Not Due to a General Medical Condition)
	787.6	Encopresis With Constipation and Overflow Incontinence
	307.7	Encopresis Without Constipation and Overflow Incontinence
	300.4	Dysthymic Disorder
	296.xx	Major Depressive Disorder

	299.80	Pervasive Developmental Disorder NOS
	309.81	Posttraumatic Stress Disorder
	308.3	Acute Stress Disorder
	_____	_____
	_____	_____
Axis II:	V71.09	No Diagnosis on Axis II
	799.9	Diagnosis Deferred
	_____	_____
	_____	_____

FIRE SETTING

BEHAVIORAL DEFINITIONS

1. One or more fires set in the last six months.
2. Fire, fireworks, or combustible substances are regularly played with.
3. Appearance wherever fire occurs.
4. Matches, lighters, candles, and so on, are consistently in his/her possession.
5. Easily discernible fascination and/or preoccupation with fire.
6. Tension or sexual arousal are not experienced prior to fire-setting behavior nor are gratification or relief when witnessing the fire.

—. _____
   _____
   _____
—. _____
   _____
   _____
—. _____
   _____

LONG-TERM GOALS

1. Secure the safety of the client, his/her family, and the community by terminating all fire-setting behavior.
2. Extinguish the client's fascination and preoccupation with fire.
3. Establish the existence of a psychotic process or major affective disorder and procure placement in an appropriate treatment program.
4. Redirect or rechannel the client's fascination with fire.

—. _____
   _____

—. _____

_____

—. _____

_____

SHORT-TERM OBJECTIVES

1. Increase the parents' ability to consistently guide and supervise the client's behavior. (1, 2, 6, 9)
2. Decrease the verbalized impulse to and actual incidence of setting fires. (3, 4, 5, 8)
3. Demonstrate the ability to safely use matches. (3, 8, 9)
4. The parents monitor the client for possessing articles connected with fire (matches, lighters, and so on). (1, 2, 4, 6)
5. The client and family members identify, express, and tolerate unpleasant feelings. (4, 10, 11, 14)
6. Increase the male client's time spent with the father or another significant male figure in his life. (4, 6, 7, 9)
7. Verbalize hurt resulting from a lack of nurturance. (6, 12, 14)
8. Verbalize feelings of anger and hurt over rejection within the family and/or from peers. (6, 12, 14)

THERAPEUTIC INTERVENTIONS

1. Assist the parents in clearly structuring and supervising the client's behavior.
2. Monitor the parents' efforts to structure, set limits on, and supervise the client, giving support, encouragement, and redirection as appropriate.
3. Assign the family an operant-based intervention (e.g., the father allows the client to strike matches under his supervision, noting the need for caution. A sum of money is placed next to the pack and the client receives a determined sum as well as warm praise for each match left unlit). The therapist monitors the intervention and gives redirection and feedback as needed.
4. Use a family systems approach to address fire-setting behavior and require the client's entire family to attend an agreed-on number of sessions, during which the family's roles, ways of communicating, and conflicts will be explored.

9. Disclose any incidents of physical or sexual abuse. (15)
10. Share memories of violent episodes that have been witnessed in the home. (13)
11. Cooperate with and evaluate the need for psychotropic medication. (16)
12. Cooperate with and complete an evaluation for ADHD. (1, 17, 18)
13. Comply with the recommendation for psychotropic medications. (1, 16, 19)

___. _____
    _____
___. _____
    _____
___. _____
    _____

5. Assist the client and his/her parents in developing ways to increase the client's impulse control through the use of positive reinforcement at times of apparent control.
6. Ask the male client's father to identify three things he could do to relate more with the client. Then assign him to implement two of the three and monitor the results.
7. Work with the client's mother or other care-giving person to obtain a Big Brother for the client.
8. Assign an intervention of stimulus satiation to preferably the father or mother (i.e., parents instruct the client how to safely strike matches, allowing the client to strike as many as he/she would like). Monitor the intervention and redirect as needed.
9. Ask the client's father in a session (or as an assignment between sessions) to teach the client how to safely build a fire, emphasizing the need for strict control of and respect for the power of fire. (The therapist provides materials in the session for fire, i.e., matches, sticks, coffee can.) The therapist monitors and processes the assignment.
10. Assist the client's family members in becoming able

to identify, express, and tolerate their own feelings and those of other family members.

11. Gently probe the client's emotions to help him/her become better able to identify and express feelings.

12. Assess the client's unmet needs for attention, nurturance, and affirmation. Urge all caregivers (parents, siblings, teachers, babysitters, and extended family) to intensify their efforts in these areas.

13. Assess the degree of chaos and/or violence in the family leading to the client's desire for power and control over his/her environment. Encourage more structure, predictability, and respect within the family.

14. Probe the client's feelings of hurt and anger over relationship rejection with his/her peers and/or the family. Interpret fire setting as an expression of rage.

15. Assess whether the client's fire setting is associated with sexual and/or physical abuse.

16. Assess whether the client's fire setting is associated with a psychotic process or major affective disorder that may need psychotropic medication treatment.

17. Assess the client for the presence of ADHD.

18. Assist the client's family in implementing the recommendations of psychiatric or ADHD evaluations.

19. Assist the family in placing the client in a residential treatment program.

___. _____

_____

___. _____

_____

___. _____

_____

DIAGNOSTIC SUGGESTIONS

Axis I:	312.81	Conduct Disorder/Childhood-Onset Type
	312.82	Conduct Disorder/Adolescent-Onset Type
	314.01	Attention-Deficit/Hyperactivity Disorder, Predominantly Hyperactive-Impulsive Type
	309.3	Adjustment Disorder With Disturbance of Conduct
	309.4	Adjustment Disorder With Mixed Disturbance of Emotions and Conduct
	312.30	Impulse Control Disorder NOS
	_____	_____
	_____	_____
Axis II:	799.9	Diagnosis Deferred
	V71.09	No Diagnosis
	_____	_____
	_____	_____

GENDER IDENTITY DISORDER

BEHAVIORAL DEFINITIONS

1. Repeatedly states the desire to be or feels he/she is the opposite sex.
2. Preference for dressing in clothes typically worn by the other sex.
3. Prefers the roles of the opposite sex in make-believe play or fantasies.
4. Insists on participating in games and pastimes that are typical of the other sex.
5. Prefers playmates of the opposite sex.
6. Frequently passes as the opposite sex.
7. Insists that he/she feels like a person of the opposite sex or was born the wrong sex.
8. Verbalizes a disgust with or rejection of his/her sexual anatomy.
9. Verbalizes the desire to be rid of primary and secondary sex characteristics through hormone or surgical procedures.

—. _____

_____

—. _____

_____

—. _____

_____

LONG-TERM GOALS

1. Terminate the confusion regarding sexual identity and accept the gender and sexual anatomy.
2. Stop dressing and playing like the opposite sex.

3. Accept the genitalia as a normal part of the body and terminate the repulsion of or desire to change it.
4. Establish and maintain a lasting (i.e., six months or longer), same-sex peer friendship.

—. _____
_____
_____

—. _____
_____
_____

—. _____
_____

SHORT-TERM OBJECTIVES

1. Openly express feelings regarding sexual identity and identify the causes for rejection of gender identity. (1, 2, 3)
2. Replace negative self-talk regarding the client's gender with positive thoughts. (4, 5)
3. Reduce the frequency of critical and repulsive statements made regarding sexual anatomy. (4, 5, 6, 7)
4. Identify positive aspects of the client's sexual role. (4, 5, 6, 7, 10)
5. Express comfort with or even pride in sexual identity. (4, 5, 6, 7)
6. The parents explore their subtle and direct messages to the client that reinforce gender identify confusion. (8, 9)

THERAPEUTIC INTERVENTIONS

1. Actively build the level of trust with the client in individual sessions through consistent eye contact, active listening, unconditional positive regard, and warm acceptance to help him/her increase the ability to identify and express feelings.
2. Explore the client's reasons for attraction to an opposite-sex identity.
3. Use play therapy techniques to explore the client's sexual attitudes and causes for the rejection of gender identity.
4. Use cognitive therapy techniques to identify and replace negative messages the client gives to him/herself about sexual identity.
5. Confront and reframe the client's self-disparaging comments about gender

7. Demonstrate increased self-esteem as evidenced by positive statements made about talents, traits, and appearance. (10, 11)

8. The same-sex parent agrees to increase contact with the client. (12, 13)

9. Verbalize the desire to be with the same-sex parent or other significant adult in quiet and active times. (12, 13)

10. The opposite-sex parent encourages and reinforces gender-appropriate dress, play, and peer group identification as well as a stronger relationship between the client and the same-sex parent. (12, 13)

11. Increase time spent in socialization with same-sex peers. (13, 14, 15)

12. Dress consistently in clothes typical of same-sex peers without objection. (12, 13, 15)

13. List some positive role models for the sexual identity and tell why they are respected. (6, 16)

14. Disclose any physical or sexual abuse. (1, 2, 3, 17)

—. _____

_____

—. _____

_____

—. _____

_____

identity and sexual anatomy.

6. Assist the client in identifying positive aspects of sexual identity.

7. Assign a mirror exercise in which the client talks positively to him/herself regarding sexual identity.

8. Hold family therapy sessions to explore the dynamics that may reinforce the client's gender confusion.

9. Meet with the parents to explore their attitudes and behaviors regarding the client's sexual identity.

10. Reinforce the client's positive self-descriptive statements.

11. Assist the client in developing a list of his/her positive traits, talents, and physical characteristics.

12. Assign the same-sex parent to increase time and contact with the client in play and work activities while urging the opposite-sex parent to support the client in appropriate identification.

13. Encourage the parents in positively reinforcing appropriate gender identity, dress, and social behavior in the client.

14. Assign the client the initiation of social (play) activities with same-sex peers.

15. Monitor and give positive feedback when the client's

dress, socialization, and peer identity are appropriate.

16. Assign the client to list some positive, same-sex role models and process reasons for respect of them.

17. Explore the possibility that the client was physically or sexually abused.

___. _____

_____

___. _____

_____

___. _____

_____

DIAGNOSTIC SUGGESTIONS

Axis I: 302.6   Gender Identity Disorder in Children
302.85   Gender Identity Disorder in Adolescents
302.6   Gender Identity Disorder NOS

_____   _____

_____   _____

Axis II: 799.9   Diagnosis Deferred
V71.09   No Diagnosis

_____   _____

_____   _____

GRIEF/LOSS UNRESOLVED

BEHAVIORAL DEFINITIONS

1. Loss of contact with a parent figure due to divorce.
2. Loss of contact with a parent figure due to the person's chronic illness or death.
3. Loss of contact with a parent figure due to termination of parental rights.
4. Loss of contact with a parent figure due to the parent's incarceration.
5. Loss of contact with a positive support network due to the client's geographic move.
6. Loss of meaningful contact with a parent figure due the parent's emotional abandonment.
7. Strong emotional response exhibited when the loss is mentioned.
8. Symptoms of lack of appetite, nightmares, restlessness, or inability to concentrate, as well as other indicators of depression that began subsequent to a loss.
9. Marked drop in school grades, increase in angry outbursts, hyperactivity, or clinginess when separating from parents, all of which are out of character for the client.
10. Feelings of guilt associated with the unreasonable belief in having done something to cause the loss or not having prevented it.
11. Avoidance of talking at length or in any depth about the loss.

___. _____
_____

___. _____
_____

___. _____
_____

LONG-TERM GOALS

1. Begin a healthy grieving process around the loss.
2. Complete the process of letting go of the lost significant other.
3. Work through the grieving and letting-go process and reach the point of emotionally reinvesting in life with joy.
4. Create a supportive emotional environment in which to successfully grieve the loss.
5. Resolve the loss and begin reinvesting in relationships with others and in age-appropriate activities.

—. _____
_____
—. _____
_____
—. _____
_____

SHORT-TERM OBJECTIVES

1. Develop a trusting relationship with the therapist as evidenced by the open communication of feelings and thoughts. (1, 2, 3)
2. Tell the story of the loss. (4, 5, 6, 7)
3. Identify feelings connected to the loss. (3, 4, 8, 9, 10)
4. Increase the ability to verbalize and experience feelings connected with the loss. (8, 9, 10)
5. Identify how the use of mood-altering substances has aided the avoidance of feelings connected to the loss. (10, 11, 12, 13)

THERAPEUTIC INTERVENTIONS

1. Actively build the level of trust with the client in individual sessions through consistent eye contact, active listening, unconditional positive regard, and warm acceptance to help increase his/her ability to identify and express feelings.
2. Educate the client and/or his/her parents on the stages of the grieving process and how to answer any questions.
3. Read with the client *Where Is Daddy?* (Goff), *Emma Says Goodbye* (Nystrom), or a similar story about loss, and afterward discuss the story.

6. Develop questions about the loss and work to obtain answers for each. (4, 10, 14)

7. Verbalize an increase in understanding of the process of grieving and letting go. (2, 7, 11, 15)

8. Identify positive things about the deceased loved one and/or the relationship and how these things may be remembered. (19, 23, 24)

9. Decrease the expression of feelings of guilt and blame for the loss. (16, 17, 18, 20)

10. Verbalize and resolve feelings of anger or guilt focused on him/herself or on the deceased loved one that block the grief process. (20, 21, 22, 25)

11. Verbalize or write a list of how the client's life will demonstrate that he/she is letting go of the loss. (13, 23, 25, 26)

12. The parents verbalize an increase in their understanding of the grief process. (27, 28, 29, 32)

13. The parents increase their verbal openness about the loss. (29, 30, 31, 32)

14. The parents identify ways to encourage and support the client in the grieving process. (28, 29, 32)

4. Work with the client in play therapy around the issues of denial and the expression of thoughts and feelings about the loss.

5. Ask the client to write a letter to the lost person describing his/her feelings and read this letter to the therapist.

6. Work with the client to tell the story of the loss by drawing pictures of his/her experience.

7. Use a mutual storytelling technique (Richard Gardner's)* in which the client tells his/her story. The therapist interprets the story for its underlying meaning and then tells a story using the same characters in a similar setting but weaves into the story a healthy way to adapt to and resolve the loss.

8. Assist the client in identifying his/her feelings by using the Five Faces Technique (*Helping Children Cope with Separation and Loss,* by Jewett).

9. Use The Ungame† to assist the client in verbalizing thoughts and feelings.

---

* R. Gardner, *Story Telling in Psychotherapy with Children* (New York: J. Aronson, 1993).
† The Ungame Co., Anaheim, California, 1984.

15. The parents who are losing custody verbally say good-bye to the client. (29, 32, 33)

16. Attend and participate in a formal session to say good-bye to the parents whose parental rights are being terminated. (34, 35)

__. _____
_____

__. _____
_____

__. _____
_____

10. Refer the client to a support group for children and adolescents from divorced families.

11. Assist the client in identifying and expressing feelings connected with the loss in individual and/or group sessions.

12. Ask the client to list ways avoidance of grieving has negatively impacted his/her life.

13. Assign the client to keep a daily grief journal of thoughts and feelings associated with the loss and how they were triggered. Share the journal in therapy sessions.

14. Assist the client in developing a list of questions about a specific loss, then find possible answers for each question.

15. Assign the client to interview a member of the clergy about death and interview an adult who has experienced the death of a loved one.

16. Explore the client's feelings of guilt and blame surrounding the loss.

17. Utilize a Despart Fable (see *Helping Children Cope with Separation and Loss* by Jewett) or a similar variation to help the client communicate blame for the loss (e.g., the therapist states: "A child says softly to him-

self, 'Oh, I am afraid.' What do you suppose the child is afraid of?").

18. Help the client lift the self-imposed curse he/she believes to be the cause for the loss by asking the person who is perceived as having imposed the curse to take it back or by using a play phone conversation for the client to apologize for the behavior which he/she believes is the cause for the curse.

19. Ask the client to write a list of positive things about the deceased and how he/she plans to remember each. Then process the list with the therapist.

20. Suggest an absolution ritual (e.g., dedicate time to a charity that the deceased loved one supported) for the client to implement to relieve the guilt or blame for the loss. Monitor the results and adjust as necessary.

21. Encourage and support the client in sessions to look angry, then act angry, and finally to put words to the anger.

22. Work with the client using behavioral techniques such as kneading clay, kicking a paper bag stuffed with newsprint, or using foam bats (Nerf Bat) to hit objects without damage in

order to release repressed feelings of anger.

23. Assign the client to write a good-bye letter to a significant other and process the letter with the therapist.

24. Ask the client to bring to a session pictures or mementos connected with the loss and talk about them with the therapist.

25. Assign the client to complete an exercise related to forgiveness and process it with the therapist in an individual session.

26. Assign the client to visit the grave of the loved one with an adult and then process the experience with the therapist.

27. Train the parents in specific ways they can provide comfort, consolation, love, companionship, and support to the client in grief.

28. Assist the parents in developing skills to help the client put feelings into words.

29. Assign the client's parents to read *Learning to Say Good-bye* (LeShan) or a similar work to help them become familiar with the grieving process.

30. Conduct family sessions where each member of the client's family talks about his/her experience related to the loss.

31. Encourage the parents to allow the client to participate in the rituals and customs of grieving if they are willing to be involved.

32. Refer the client's parents to a grief/loss support group.

33. Conduct a session with the parents who are losing custody of the client to prepare him/her to say good-bye to the client in a healthy, affirming way.

34. Assist the client in making a record of his/her life in a book format to help visualize the past, present, and future life. When it is completed, the client keeps a copy and gives another to the current parents.

35. Facilitate a good-bye session with the client and the parents who are losing custody, for the purpose of giving the client permission to move on with his/her life. If parents who are losing custody or current parents are not available, ask them to write a letter that can be read at the session or conduct a role play in which the client says good-bye to each parent.

__. _____
   _____

__. _____
   _____

__. _____
   _____

DIAGNOSTIC SUGGESTIONS

Axis I:

296.2x	Major Depressive Disorder, Single Episode
296.3x	Major Depressive Disorder, Recurrent
V62.82	Bereavement
309.0	Adjustment Disorder With Depressed Mood
309.4	Adjustment Disorder With Mixed Disturbance of Emotions and Conduct
300.4	Dysthymic Disorder
_____	_____
_____	_____

Axis II:

799.9	Diagnosis Deferred
V71.09	No Diagnosis
_____	_____
_____	_____

LEARNING DISORDER/ UNDERACHIEVEMENT

BEHAVIORAL DEFINITIONS

1. Reading achievement, as measured by individually administered, standardized tests of reading recognition or comprehension, is significantly below the expected level, given the client's chronological age, grade, and measured intelligence.
2. Mathematical ability, as measured by individually administered, standardized tests, is significantly below the expected level, given the client's chronological age, grade, and measured intelligence.
3. Writing skills, as measured by individually administered, standardized tests, are significantly below the expected level given the client's chronological age, grade, and measured intelligence.
4. History of overall academic performance that is below that expected, given the client's measured intelligence.
5. Learning disability substantially interferes with the client's academic performance or activities of daily living that require any or all of the following academic skills: reading, mathematics, and written expression.
6. Feelings of low self-esteem, depression, and anxiety, which arise from the learning disability, further exacerbate learning problems.
7. Recurrent pattern of engaging in acting-out, disruptive, and negative attention-seeking behaviors when encountering difficulty or frustration in learning.
8. Positive family history of members having academic difficulties, disinterest, or failures.

—. _____

_____

—. _____
_____
—. _____
_____

LONG-TERM GOALS

1. Demonstrate consistent interest, initiative, and motivation in academics and bring the performance level up to that expected for intellectual ability.
2. Achieve the academic goals identified on the client's Individualized Educational Plan (IEP).
3. Perform to the level of capability in the area of academic weakness.
4. Develop an awareness and acceptance of the learning disability so that the client is able to maintain a healthy balance between accomplishing academic goals and meeting his/her social, emotional, and self-esteem needs.
5. Build self-esteem so that the client is able to cope effectively with the frustrations associated with the learning disability and complete school or homework assignments on a consistent basis without giving up.
6. Eliminate the pattern of engaging in acting-out, disruptive, or negative attention-seeking behaviors when confronted with difficulty or frustration in learning.
7. Parents establish realistic expectations of the client's learning abilities and implement effective intervention strategies at home to help the client keep up with schoolwork and achieve academic goals.
8. Remove emotional impediments or resolve family conflicts that will allow for improved academic achievement.

—. _____
_____
—. _____
_____
—. _____
_____

SHORT-TERM OBJECTIVES

1. Complete a psychoeducational evaluation. (1, 3, 4)
2. Complete psychological testing. (2, 4, 34)
3. The client and his/her parents provide psychosocial history information. (3, 4)
4. Cooperate with a hearing, vision, or medical examination. (5, 34)
5. Comply with the recommendations made by the multidisciplinary evaluation team at school regarding educational interventions. (1, 2, 6, 7)
6. Move the client to an appropriate classroom setting(s). (1, 6, 9, 10)
7. Complete neuropsychological testing. (6, 8)
8. Parents and teachers implement educational strategies that maximize the child's learning strengths and compensate for learning weaknesses. (7, 8, 9, 10)
9. Participate in outside tutoring to increase knowledge and skills in the area of academic weakness. (9, 11, 12)
10. Cooperate with the recommendations offered by the private learning center. (10, 11, 12)
11. Implement effective study skills, which increase the frequency of completion of school assignments and

THERAPEUTIC INTERVENTIONS

1. Arrange for psychoeducational testing to evaluate the presence of a learning disability and determine whether the client is eligible to receive special education services.
2. Arrange for psychological testing to assess whether a possible ADHD or emotional factors are interfering with the client's learning abilities.
3. Gather psychosocial history information that includes key developmental milestones and a family history of educational achievements and failures.
4. Provide feedback to the client, his/her family, and school officials regarding psychoeducational and/or psychological evaluation.
5. Refer the client for hearing, vision, or medical examination to rule out possible hearing, visual, or health problems that are interfering with learning abilities.
6. Attend an Individualized Educational Planning Committee (IEPC) meeting with the parents, teachers, and school officials to determine the client's eligibility for special education services, design educational interventions, and establish educational goals.

improve academic performance. (7, 11, 13, 16)

12. Develop effective test-taking strategies, which decrease anxiety and improve test performance. (10, 11, 12, 16)

13. The parents maintain regular communication (i.e., daily to weekly) with teachers. (7, 13, 16)

14. Establish a regular routine that allows time to engage in play, spend quality time with the family, and complete homework assignments. (11, 16)

15. Increase praise and positive reinforcement by the parents toward the client in regard to school performance. (13, 17, 21)

16. Identify and remove all emotional blocks or learning inhibitions that are within the client and/or the family system. (14, 15)

17. The parents verbally identify their denial of the client's learning disability and how it interferes with learning progress. (14, 15, 19, 20)

18. Cease denial in the family system about the client's learning disability. (19, 20, 25)

19. Increase the parents' time spent involved with the client's homework. (15, 17, 20, 21)

20. The parents verbally acknowledge their unrealis-

7. Consult with the client, parents, and school officials about designing effective learning programs or intervention strategies that build on the client's strengths and compensate for weaknesses.

8. Arrange for neuropsychological testing to rule out the presence of neurological/organic factors contributing to the learning problem.

9. Recommend that the parents seek outside tutoring after school to boost the client's skills in the area of his/her academic weakness (i.e., reading, mathematics, or written expression).

10. Refer the client to a private learning center for extra tutoring in the areas of academic weakness and assistance in improving study and test-taking skills.

11. Teach the client more effective study skills (e.g., remove distractions, study in quiet places, develop outlines, highlight important details, schedule breaks).

12. Teach the client more effective test-taking strategies (e.g., study over an extended period of time, review material regularly, read directions twice, recheck work).

13. Encourage the parents to maintain regular (daily or weekly) communication with teachers to help the

tic expectations or excessive pressure on the client to perform. (14, 15, 22, 23, 26)

21. The parents verbally recognize that their pattern of overprotectiveness interferes with the client's academic growth and responsibility. (14, 15, 24, 25)

22. Increase the frequency of on-task behavior at school, increasing the completion of school assignments without expressing frustration and the desire to give up. (18, 27, 28, 30, 32)

23. Increase the frequency of positive statements about school experiences and confidence in the ability to succeed academically. (18, 27, 29, 30, 31, 32)

24. Decrease the frequency and severity of acting-out behaviors when encountering frustration with school assignments. (18, 28, 32, 33, 34)

25. Take prescribed medication as directed by the physician. (2, 34)

___. _____
_____

___. _____
_____

___. _____
_____

client remain organized and keep up with school assignments.

14. Conduct family sessions that probe the client's family system to identify any emotional block or inhibitions to learning.

15. Assist the parents in resolving family conflicts that block or inhibit learning and establish new positive family patterns that reinforce the client's academic achievement.

16. Assist the client and his/her parents in developing a routine daily schedule at home that allows the client to achieve a healthy balance of completing school/homework assignments, engaging in independent play, and spending quality time with family and peers.

17. Encourage the parents to give frequent praise and positive reinforcement for the client's effort and accomplishment on academic tasks.

18. Assist the client's parents and teachers in the development of systematic rewards for progress and accomplishments (e.g., charts with stars for goal attainment, praise for each success, some material reward for achievement).

19. Educate the client's parents about the signs and symptoms of learning disabilities.

20. Confront, challenge, and work through the parents' denial surrounding the client's learning disability so that they cooperate with recommendations regarding placement and educational interventions.

21. Encourage the parents to demonstrate and/or maintain regular interest and involvement in the client's homework (i.e., the parents read aloud or alongside the client, use flash cards to improve math skills, recheck the client's spelling words).

22. Conduct family therapy sessions to assess whether the parents have developed unrealistic expectations or are placing excessive pressure on the client to perform.

23. Confront and challenge the parents about placing excessive pressure on the client.

24. Observe parent-child interactions to assess whether the parents' overprotectiveness or infantilization of the client contributes to his/her academic underachievement.

25. Assist the parents in developing realistic expectations of the client's learning potential.

26. Assist the client in coming to an understanding and acceptance of the limitations surrounding the learning disability.

27. Consult with school officials about ways to improve the client's on-task behaviors (e.g., keep the client close to the teacher, keep the client close to positive peer role models, call on the client often, provide frequent feedback to the client, structure the material into a series of small steps).

28. Teach the client positive coping mechanisms (e.g., relaxation techniques, positive self-talk, cognitive restructuring) to utilize when encountering frustration or difficulty with schoolwork.

29. Reinforce the client's successful school experiences and positive statements about school.

30. Confront the client's self-disparaging remarks and expressed desire to give up on school assignments.

31. Assign the client the task of making one positive self-statement daily about school and his/her ability and recording it in a journal.

32. Help the client identify what rewards would increase his/her motivation to improve academic performance and then implement the suggestions into the academic program.

33. Teach the client positive coping and self-control strategies (e.g., cognitive restructuring, positive self-

talk, "stop, look, listen, and think") to inhibit the impulse to act out or engage in negative attention-seeking behaviors when encountering frustration with schoolwork.

34. Arrange for a medication evaluation of the client if it is determined that an emotional problem and/or ADHD are interfering with learning.

—. _____

_____

—. _____

_____

—. _____

_____

DIAGNOSTIC SUGGESTIONS

Axis I:	315.0	Learning Disorder
	315.1	Mathematics Disorder
	315.2	Disorder of Written Expression
	315.9	Learning Disorder NOS
	V62.3	Academic Problem
	314.01	Attention-Deficit/Hyperactivity Disorder, Combined Type
	314.00	Attention-Deficit/Hyperactivity Disorder, Predominantly Inattentive Type
	300.4	Dysthymic Disorder
	_____	_____
	_____	_____
Axis II:	317.	Mild Mental Retardation
	V62.89	Borderline Intellectual Functioning
	799.9	Diagnosis Deferred
	V71.09	No Diagnosis
	_____	_____
	_____	_____

LOW SELF-ESTEEM

BEHAVIORAL DEFINITIONS

1. Inability to accept compliments.
2. Verbalization of self-disparaging remarks; seeing him/herself as unattractive, worthless, stupid, a loser, a burden, and unimportant; taking blame easily.
3. Avoiding contact with adults and peers.
4. Excessively seeking to please or receive attention and praise from adults and/or peers.
5. Inability to identify or accept his/her positive traits or talents.
6. Fear of rejection by others, especially the peer group.
7. Acting out in negative ways that are quite obviously attention seeking.
8. Difficulty saying no to others; fear of not being liked by others.

—. _____
_____
_____

—. _____
_____
_____

—. _____
_____

LONG-TERM GOALS

1. Elevate self-esteem.
2. Continue to build a consistent positive self-image.
3. Demonstrate improved self-esteem through accepting compliments, identifying positive characteristics about him/herself, being able to say no to others, and the absence of self-disparaging remarks.

4. Attain the core belief that he/she is lovable and capable.

—. _____

   _____

—. _____

   _____

—. _____

   _____

SHORT-TERM OBJECTIVES

1. Verbalize an increased awareness of self-disparaging statements. (1, 2, 4, 10)
2. Decrease the frequency of negative self-descriptive statements. (2, 4, 5, 6)
3. Decrease the verbalized fear of rejection while increasing statements of self-acceptance. (3, 5, 6, 8)
4. Identify positive traits and talents about him/herself. (4, 5, 6, 7)
5. Develop the ability to identify and verbalize feelings. (4, 5, 11, 12)
6. Increase eye contact with others. (4, 9, 10)
7. Identify accomplishments that can improve self-image. (4, 11, 14, 15)
8. Develop the ability to identify and express verbally his/her needs. (4, 16, 17, 18)

THERAPEUTIC INTERVENTIONS

1. Confront and reframe the client's self-disparaging comments.
2. Assist the client in becoming aware of how he/she expresses or acts out negative feelings about him/herself.
3. Probe the parents' interactions with the client in family sessions and redirect or rechannel any patterns of interaction or methods of discipline that are demeaning of the patient.
4. Refer the client to a self-esteem group.
5. Ask the client to make one positive statement about him/herself daily and record it on a chart or in a journal.
6. Assist the client in developing self-talk as a way of boosting his/her confidence and positive self-image.

9. Show recognition verbally or in writing of the secondary gains received from negative behaviors. (4, 11, 23, 24)

10. Take responsibility for daily self-care tasks that are developmentally age appropriate. (4, 11, 21)

11. List specific things he/she can do to build self-esteem and ways to implement each. (4, 11, 15, 18)

12. Positively acknowledge and verbally accept praise or compliments from others. (4, 10, 15, 24)

13. Develop positive self-talk messages to build self-esteem. (4, 6, 11, 15)

14. The parents identify specific ways they can assist in developing self-esteem in the client. (17, 21, 25, 26, 27)

15. The parents verbalize realistic expectations for the client. (25, 26, 28)

16. The parents verbally reinforce the client's active attempts to build self-esteem. (17, 25, 26)

17. Increase the frequency of speaking up with confidence in social situations. (4, 15, 18, 20)

7. Develop with the client a list of affirmations and have him/her read it three times a day to him/herself.

8. Reinforce verbally the client's use of statements of confidence or positive evaluation about him/herself.

9. Assist the client in making consistent eye contact with whomever he/she is speaking.

10. Ask the client to make eye contact when speaking to the therapist during a session, to teachers at school, and to parents at home.

11. Assign self-esteem-building exercises from a workbook such as *The Building Blocks of Self-Esteem* (Shapiro) or a selected individual exercise.

12. Use a therapeutic game such as Talking, Feeling, Doing* or The Ungame[†] to promote the client's awareness of him/herself and his/her feelings.

13. Educate the client in the basics of feelings and assist him/her in beginning to identify them.

14. Use play therapy techniques to probe the causes for the client's low self-esteem.

---

* Creative Therapeutics, Cresskill, New Jersey, 1973.
[†] The Ungame Co., Anaheim, California, 1984.

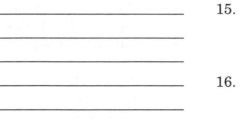

——. _____

——. _____

——. _____

15. Use role play and behavioral rehearsal to improve the client's assertiveness and social skills.

16. Assist the client in becoming capable of identifying and verbalizing needs.

17. Conduct a family session in which the client expresses his/her needs to the family and vice versa.

18. Use therapeutic stories (Gardner)* to help the client identify feelings and needs and to build self-esteem.

19. Use neurolinguistic programming (NLP) or reframing techniques in which messages about the self are changed to enhance the client's self-esteem.

20. Help the client reduce the fear of rejections.

21. Help the client and his/her family identify and implement daily responsibilities for the client that are age appropriate. Monitor the follow-through and give positive verbal feedback when warranted.

22. Discuss and interpret incidents of abuse (emotional, physical, sexual) as to how they have impacted the client's feelings about him/herself.

---

* R. Gardner, *Fairy Tales for Today's Children* (Cresskill, New Jersey: Creative Therapeutics, 1978).

23. Help the client identify distorted negative beliefs about him/herself and the world.

24. Reinforce the client's use of more realistic, positive messages to him/herself in interpreting life events.

25. Ask the client's parents to attend a series on positive parenting; then process how they can implement some of these techniques.

26. Assist the parents in developing and implementing specific ways to boost the client's self-esteem.

27. Ask the parents to involve the client in activities that are self-esteem-building, such as scouting, experiential camps, music, sports, youth groups, and enrichment programs.

28. Explore the parents' expectations of the client and assist, if necessary, in making them more realistic.

__. _____
   _____

__. _____
   _____

__. _____
   _____

DIAGNOSTIC SUGGESTIONS

Axis I:

300.4	Dysthymic Disorder
314.01	Attention-Deficit/Hyperactivity Disorder, Predominantly Hyperactive-Impulsive Type
300.23	Social Phobia
266.xx	Major Depressive Disorder
309.21	Separation Anxiety
300.02	Generalized Anxiety
V61.21	Physical Abuse of Child, 995.54 Victim
V61.21	Sexual Abuse of Child, 995.53 Victim
V61.21	Neglect of Child, 995.52 Victim
303.90	Alcohol Dependence
304.30	Cannabis Dependence
_____	_____
_____	_____

Axis II:

317.00	Mild Mental Retardation
V62.89	Borderline Intellectual Functioning
799.9	Diagnosis Deferred
V71.09	No Diagnosis
_____	_____
_____	_____

MANIA/HYPOMANIA

BEHAVIORAL DEFINITIONS

1. Loud, overly friendly social style that oversteps social boundaries and shows poor social judgment (e.g., too trusting and self-disclosing too quickly).
2. Inflated sense of self-esteem and an exaggerated, euphoric belief in capabilities that denies any self-limitations or realistic obstacles but sees others as standing in the way.
3. Flighty thoughts.
4. Pressured speech.
5. High energy and restlessness.
6. Disorganized impulsivity that does not foresee the consequences of the behavior.
7. A reduced need for sleep and a denial of emotional or physical pain.
8. A positive family history of affective disorder.
9. Verbal and/or physical aggression coupled with tantrumlike behavior (e.g., breaking things explosively) if wishes are blocked, which is in contrast to an earlier pattern of obedience and restraint.
10. Poor attention span and susceptibility to distraction.
11. Lack of follow-through in projects even though the energy level is very high, since the behavior lacks discipline and goal-directedness.
12. Impulsive behaviors that reflect a lack of recognition of self-defeating consequences (e.g., shoplifting, alcohol abuse, drug abuse, or sexual promiscuity).
13. Outlandish dress and grooming.

—. _____
_____
—. _____
_____

—. _____
_____

LONG-TERM GOALS

1. Increase the control over impulses, reduce the energy level, and stabilize the mood.
2. Decrease irritability and impulsivity, improve social judgment, and develop a sensitivity to the consequences of behavior while having more realistic expectations of him/herself.
3. Acknowledge the underlying depression and cope with feelings or fear of loss.
4. Talk about underlying feelings of low self-esteem or guilt and fears of rejection, dependency, and abandonment by significant others.

—. _____
_____

—. _____
_____

—. _____
_____

SHORT-TERM OBJECTIVES

1. Take psychotropic medications as directed. (1, 2, 3)
2. Begin to demonstrate trust in the therapy relationship by sharing fears about dependency, loss, and abandonment. (4, 5, 6, 9)
3. Achieve mood stability, becoming slower to react with anger, less expansive, and more socially appropriate and sensitive. (11, 15, 16, 21)

THERAPEUTIC INTERVENTIONS

1. Assess the client's need for mood-stabilizing medication (e.g., lithium carbonate).
2. Arrange for a medication prescription to aid the client in reducing euphoric energy.
3. Monitor the client's reaction to the medication (i.e., side effects and effectiveness).
4. Pledge to be there consistently to help, listen to, and support the client.
5. Explore the client's fears of abandonment by sources of love and nurturance.

4. Verbalize grief, fear, and anger regarding real or imagined losses in life. (5, 6, 7, 8)

5. Acknowledge the low self-esteem and fear of rejection that underlie the braggadocio. (9, 10, 11, 12)

6. Identify the causes for the low self-esteem and abandonment fears. (9, 10, 12)

7. Differentiate between real and imagined losses, rejections, and abandonments. (6, 8)

8. The parents reinforce positive behaviors while setting firm limits on hostility. (10, 11, 19, 21, 22)

9. Terminate self-destructive behaviors such as promiscuity, substance abuse, and the expression of overt hostility or aggression. (13, 15, 16)

10. Speak more slowly and be more subject-focused. (13, 14)

11. Dress and groom in a less attention-seeking manner. (11, 18, 20)

12. Verbalize the acceptance of and peace with dependency needs. (4, 5, 10, 18)

13. Identify positive traits and behaviors that build genuine self-esteem. (19, 20)

14. Decrease grandiose statements and express him/herself more realistically. (11, 15, 17)

6. Probe real or perceived losses in the client's life.

7. Review ways to replace the losses and put them in perspective.

8. Help the client differentiate between real and imagined, actual and exaggerated losses.

9. Probe the causes for the client's low self-esteem and abandonment fears in the family-of-origin history.

10. Hold family therapy sessions to explore and confront parental rejection or emotional abandonment.

11. Confront the client's grandiosity and demandingness gradually but firmly.

12. Explore the stressors that precipitate the client's manic behavior (e.g., school failure, social rejection, family trauma).

13. Provide structure and focus for the client's thoughts and actions by regulating the direction of conversation and establishing plans for behavior.

14. Verbally reinforce slower speech and more deliberate thought processes.

15. Repeatedly focus on the consequences of behavior to reduce thoughtless impulsivity.

16. Facilitate impulse control by using role play, behavior rehearsal, and role reversal

15. Identify stressors that increase the fear of rejection and failure. (12, 17, 18)

16. Accept the limits set on manipulative and hostile behaviors that attempt to control others. (21, 22)

___. _____
    _____
___. _____
    _____
___. _____
    _____

to increase sensitivity to the consequences of behavior.

17. Encourage the client to share feelings at a deeper level to facilitate openness, intimacy, and trust in relationships and counteract denial, fear, and superficiality.

18. Interpret the fear and insecurity underlying the client's braggadocio, hostility, and denial of dependency.

19. Assist the client in identifying strengths and assets to build self-esteem and confidence.

20. Encourage and reinforce appropriate dress and grooming.

21. Set limits on manipulation or acting out by making rules and establishing clear consequences for breaking them.

22. Reinforce the parents in setting reasonable limits on the client's behavior and in expressing their commitment to love him/her unconditionally.

___. _____
    _____
___. _____
    _____
___. _____
    _____

DIAGNOSTIC SUGGESTIONS

Axis I: 296.xx   Bipolar I Disorder
296.89   Bipolar II Disorder
301.13   Cyclothymic Disorder
295.70   Schizoaffective Disorder
296.80   Bipolar Disorder NOS
310.1   Personality Change Due to (Axis III Disorder)
314.01   Attention-Deficit/Hyperactivity Disorder,
Predominantly Hyperactive-Impulsive Type

_____   _____

_____   _____

Axis II: 799.9   Diagnosis Deferred
V71.09   No Diagnosis

_____   _____

_____   _____

MENTAL RETARDATION

BEHAVIORAL DEFINITIONS

1. Significantly subaverage intellectual functioning as demonstrated by an IQ score of approximately 70 or below on an individually administered intelligence test.
2. Significant impairments in communication, self-care, home living, social skills, self-direction, use of community resources, academic skills, work, and leisure.
3. Difficulty understanding and following complex directions at home, in school, and in vocational settings.
4. Short- and long-term memory impairment.
5. Concrete thinking or impaired abstract reasoning abilities.
6. Impoverished social skills as manifested by frequent use of poor judgment and limited understanding of the antecedents and consequences of social actions or nuances.
7. Lack of insight and repeated failure to learn from experience or past mistakes.
8. Low self-esteem as evidenced by frequent self-derogatory remarks (e.g., "I am so stupid").
9. Recurrent pattern of acting without considering the consequences of the actions.

__. _____
   _____

__. _____
   _____

__. _____
   _____

LONG-TERM GOALS

1. Achieve all academic goals identified on the client's Individualized Educational Plan (IEP).
2. Achieve all behavioral, social-interpersonal, self-care, and home living goals identified on the client's Individual Service Plan.
3. Function at an appropriate level of independence in residential, educational, and vocational settings.
4. Develop an awareness and acceptance of intellectual and cognitive limitations so that the client can consistently verbalize feelings of self-worth.
5. Parents and/or caregivers develop an awareness and acceptance of the client's intellectual and cognitive capabilities so that they place appropriate expectations on his/her functioning.
6. Consistently comply and follow through with a daily routine and simple directions at home, in school, or in a vocational setting.
7. Reduce the frequency and severity of socially inappropriate behaviors.

—. _____
   _____
—. _____
   _____
—. _____
   _____

SHORT-TERM OBJECTIVES

1. Complete a comprehensive intellectual and cognitive assessment. (1, 4, 7)
2. Complete psychological testing. (2, 4, 7)
3. Complete neuropsychological testing. (3, 4, 7)
4. Complete an evaluation by physical and occupational therapists. (5, 7)

THERAPEUTIC INTERVENTIONS

1. Arrange for a comprehensive intellectual and cognitive assessment to determine the presence of mental retardation and gain greater insight into the client's learning strengths and weaknesses.
2. Arrange for psychological testing to assess whether emotional factors or ADHD are interfering with the

5. Complete a speech/language evaluation. (6, 7)

6. The client and his/her parents comply with recommendations made by a multidisciplinary evaluation team at school regarding educational interventions. (7, 8)

7. Move the client to appropriate classroom(s) in a school setting or residential program. (7, 9, 10)

8. Move the client to an appropriate residential setting. (8, 9)

9. The client's parents and teachers implement educational strategies that maximize his/her learning strengths and compensate for learning weaknesses. (7, 8, 11, 12)

10. Receive appropriate auxiliary services (e.g., physical, speech/language, occupational therapy, and counseling). (5, 6, 7, 10)

11. The client's parents maintain regular communication with his/her teachers and other appropriate school officials. (8, 11, 14)

12. Implement a token economy in the classroom or placement setting to reinforce on-task behaviors, completion of school assignments, good impulse control, and positive social skills. (11, 12, 13)

client's intellectual and academic functioning.

3. Arrange for a neurological examination or neuropsychological testing to rule out possible organic factors that may be contributing to the client's intellectual or cognitive deficits.

4. Provide feedback to the client, his/her parents, school officials, and residential staff regarding the intellectual, psychological, or neuropsychological testing.

5. Refer the client to physical and occupational therapists to assess perceptual or sensory-motor deficits and determine the need for ongoing physical and/or occupational therapy.

6. Refer the client to a speech/language pathologist to assess deficits and determine the need for appropriate therapy.

7. Attend an Individualized Educational Planning Committee meeting with the client's parents, teachers, and other appropriate professionals to determine his/her eligibility for special education services, design educational interventions, and establish goals.

8. Consult with the client, his/her parents, teachers, and other appropriate school officials about designing effective learning

13. Increase the parent's praise and other positive reinforcement toward the client in regard to his/her academic performance or social behaviors. (13, 14)

14. Agree to and implement a contingency contract with the client, his/her parents, and teachers to improve academic performance, deter impulsive behaviors, and increase positive social behaviors. (11, 13, 14)

15. Cease verbalizations of denial in the family system about the client's intellectual and cognitive deficits. (15, 16)

16. The parents recognize and verbally acknowledge their unrealistic expectations of or excessive pressure on the client to function at an unrealistic level. (15, 17, 18, 20)

17. The parents recognize and verbally acknowledge that their pattern of overprotectiveness interferes with the client's intellectual, emotional, and social development. (15, 19, 20, 21)

18. Reduce the frequency of the parents speaking for the client or performing activities that he/she is capable of doing independently. (19, 20, 21, 22)

19. Increase the client's participation in family activities, outings, or responsibilities. (21, 22, 23, 26)

programs or interventions that build on the client's strengths and compensate for weaknesses.

9. Consult with the client's parents, school officials, or mental health professionals about the need for placement in a foster home, group home, or residential program.

10. Refer the client to a sheltered workshop or educational rehabilitation center to develop basic job skills.

11. Encourage the parents to maintain regular communication with the client's teacher or school officials to monitor his/her academic, behavioral, emotional, and social progress.

12. Design a token economy for the classroom or residential program to improve the client's academic performance, impulse control, and social skills.

13. Encourage the client's parents to provide frequent praise and other reinforcement for positive social behaviors and academic performance.

14. Design a reward system or contingency contract to reinforce desired adaptive or social behaviors.

15. Educate the client's parents about the symptoms and characteristics of mental retardation.

20. The parents implement behavior management techniques to reduce the frequency and severity of temper outbursts and aggressive behaviors. (24, 25, 28)

21. The client and his/her parents agree to and implement an allowance program that helps the client learn to manage money more effectively. (20, 26)

22. Take a bath or shower, comb hair, brush teeth, and apply deodorant daily. (20, 27)

23. Initiate appropriate social greetings, smile, and make eye contact when entering a social situation. (29, 30)

24. Increase the frequency of positive self-statements by the client. (31, 32)

25. Increase the client's ability to identify and express feelings. (33, 34)

26. Recognize and verbally identify appropriate and inappropriate sexual behaviors. (28, 35)

27. Take medication as prescribed by the physician. (2, 3, 36)

___. _____
    _____

___. _____
    _____

___. _____
    _____

16. Confront and challenge the parents' denial surrounding their child's intellectual deficits so they cooperate with recommendations regarding placement and educational interventions.

17. Conduct family therapy sessions to assess whether the parents are placing excessive pressure on the client to function at level that he/she is not capable of achieving.

18. Confront and challenge the parents about placing excessive pressure on the client.

19. Observe parent-child interactions to assess whether the parents' overprotectiveness or infantilization of the client interferes with his/her intellectual, emotional, or social development.

20. Assist the client's parents or caregivers in developing realistic expectations of his/her intellectual capabilities and level of adaptive functioning.

21. Encourage the client's parents and family members to regularly include the patient in outings or activities (e.g., attend sporting events, go ice skating, visit a child's museum).

22. Assign the client a task in the family (e.g., cooking a simple meal, gardening) that is appropriate for

his/her level of functioning and provides him/her with a sense of responsibility or belonging.

23. Consult with school officials or residential staff about the client performing a job (e.g., raise the flag, help run video equipment) to build self-esteem and provide him/her with a sense of responsibility.

24. Teach the parents effective behavior management techniques (i.e., time-outs, removal of privileges) to decrease the frequency and severity of the client's temper outbursts, acting out, and aggressive behaviors.

25. Encourage the parents to utilize natural, logical consequences for the client's inappropriate social or maladaptive behaviors.

26. Counsel the parents about setting up an allowance plan which seeks to increase the client's responsibilities and help him/her learn simple money management skills.

27. Design a reward system at home to improve the client's personal hygiene and self-help skills.

28. Teach the client basic mediational and self-control strategies (e.g., "stop, look, listen, and think") to delay gratification and inhibit impulses.

29. Identify and reinforce the client's positive social behaviors.

30. Utilize role play, modeling, and puppets in individual sessions to improve the client's social skills.

31. Encourage the client to participate in the Special Olympics to build self-esteem.

32. Assist the client in coming to an understanding and acceptance of the limitations surrounding his/her intellectual deficits and adaptive functioning.

33. Teach the client effective communication skills (i.e., proper listening, good eye contact, "I" statements) to improve his/her ability to express thoughts, feelings, and needs more clearly.

34. Educate the client about different emotions.

35. Provide sex education to help the client identify and verbally recognize appropriate and inappropriate sexual behaviors.

36. Arrange for a medication evaluation of the client.

__. _____

_____

__. _____

_____

__. _____

_____

DIAGNOSTIC SUGGESTIONS

Axis I: 299.00   Autistic Disorder
299.80   Rett's Disorder
299.8   Asperger's Disorder
299.10   Childhood Disintegrative Disorder

_____   _____

_____   _____

Axis II: 317   Mild Mental Retardation
318.0   Moderate Mental Retardation
318.1   Severe Mental Retardation
318.2   Profound Mental Retardation
319.1   Mental Retardation, Severity Unspecified
V62.89   Borderline Intellectual Functioning
799.9   Diagnosis Deferred
V71.09   No Diagnosis

_____   _____

_____   _____

OPPOSITIONAL DEFIANT

BEHAVIORAL DEFINITIONS

1. Pattern of negativistic, hostile, and defiant behavior toward all adults.
2. Acting as if parents, teachers, and other authority figures are the enemy.
3. Temper tantrums (e.g., screaming, crying, throwing objects, thrashing on ground, or refusing to move) in defiance of direction from an adult caregiver.
4. Constant arguing with adults.
5. Defying or refusing to comply with requests and rules even when they are reasonable.
6. Deliberate annoyance of people and susceptibility to annoyance from others.
7. Blaming others for his/her mistakes or misbehavior.
8. Consistent display of anger and resentment.
9. Frequent display of spite or vindictiveness.
10. Significant impairment in social, academic, or occupational functioning due to obstreperous behavior.

—. _____
_____

—. _____
_____

—. _____
_____

LONG-TERM GOALS

1. Markedly reduce the intensity and frequency of hostile and defiant behavior toward adults.
2. Terminate temper tantrums and replace them with calm, respectful compliance with adult directions.
3. Begin to consistently interact with adults in a mutually respectful manner.
4. Bring hostile, defiant behavior within socially acceptable standards.
5. Replace hostile, defiant behavior toward adults with respect and cooperation.
6. Resolve the conflict that underlies the anger, hostility, and defiance.
7. Reach a level of reduced tension, increased satisfaction, and improved communication between the client and his/her family.

—. _____

_____

—. _____

_____

—. _____

_____

SHORT-TERM OBJECTIVES

1. Develop a working relationship with the therapist in which the client shares his/her thoughts and feelings openly. (1, 2, 6)

2. Decrease the frequency and intensity of hostile, negativistic, and defiant interactions with parents and other adults. (1, 2, 3, 4)

3. Identify how the client would like to be treated by his/her parents and other adults. (1, 4, 8)

THERAPEUTIC INTERVENTIONS

1. Actively build the level of trust with the client in individual sessions through consistent eye contact, active listening, unconditional positive regard, and warm acceptance to help increase his/her ability to identify and express feelings.

2. Encourage the client to verbalize in individual sessions the sources of negative, hostile feelings in an open, accepting, and understanding manner.

4. Increase the client's ability to recognize and verbalize hurt or angry feelings in constructive ways. (1, 2, 5, 6)

5. Develop the ability to verbalize the connection between feelings and behavior. (2, 5, 6, 7)

6. Increase the ability to identify and verbalize what he/she needs from the parents or other adults. (4, 5, 6, 7)

7. Increase the frequency of civil, respectful interactions between the client and his/her parents or other adults. (7, 8, 9)

8. Identify angry feelings, the object of the anger, and the reasons for it. (5, 6, 7, 17)

9. Show verbal recognition of what is acceptable and unacceptable behavior in the family and the consequence of being exiled unless the behavior is kept within these limits. (9, 10, 11, 12)

10. The client and his/her parents reinforce each other positively and ignore inappropriate behaviors. (9, 12, 13, 15)

11. The parents develop clear boundaries and behavioral expectations for the client and implement specific con-

3. Process with the client his/her negative, hostile, and defiant behaviors and then offer a paradoxical interpretation or reframing for each (e.g., "Do you want Mom to put you in time-out more often?").

4. Facilitate family therapy sessions in which the issues of respect, cooperation, and conflict resolution are addressed and possible solutions are reached and implemented.

5. Assist the client in becoming able to recognize feelings and express them in constructive, respectful ways.

6. Use a therapeutic game (Talking, Feeling, Doing* or The Ungame†) to expand the client's self-awareness.

7. Probe the feelings associated with defiance to help the client make connections between feelings and behaviors.

8. Review with the client the basics of treating others respectfully. Then ask him/her to treat everyone in a respectful manner for one week. Monitor and process the experience.

9. Videotape a family session, using appropriate portions to show the destructive family interaction patterns and

---

* Creative Therapeutics, Cresskill, New Jersey, 1973.
† The Ungame Co., Anaheim, California, 1984.

sequences when any are violated as well as rewards when they are respected. (9, 12, 18, 19)

12. The parents provide corrective social interaction for the client. (12, 13, 16, 18)

13. The parents develop, implement, and administer a behavior modification contract with the client. (11, 12, 13, 19)

14. The client and his/her family comply by implementing the strategic, structural, or other directives prescribed by the therapist. (14, 15, 21, 22)

—. _____

    _____

—. _____

    _____

—. _____

    _____

to develop more respectful patterns to implement.

10. Help the parents clarify and communicate to the client what is acceptable and unacceptable behavior in the family. Then implement a consequence of temporary exile from the family (i.e., withdrawal of interactions and privileges when unacceptable behavior is exhibited). Interaction and privileges are instituted only as a result of acceptable behavior.

11. Conduct family sessions during which the therapist models child-rearing techniques for the client's parents.

12. Instruct the parents to reduce their own unproductive ororverbalizations to the client, ignore abusive/negative behaviors, and use positive and negative reinforcement techniques.

13. Monitor the parents' use of the new reinforcement techniques, giving feedback and suggesting adjustments as needed.

14. Facilitate a family session in which the family is sculpted as they are (Satir).* Process the experience with the family, then sculpt them as they would like to be.

---

* V. Satir, *Peoplemaking* (Palo Alto, California: Science and Behavior Books, 1972), pp. 154–170.

15. Conduct a family session in which the family is given a task or problem to solve together (a craft or an exercise such as making a coat of arms or a collage). Observe and then process what the experience was like for them.

16. Focus the family sessions on any marital or parenting conflict that underlies the client's behavior. Work with his/her parents in conjoint sessions to begin to resolve their issues.

17. Use a family-systems approach in individual sessions with the client to assist in understanding the family from a different perspective and move him/her toward disengaging from the dysfunctional family dynamics.

18. Assist the parents in defining acceptable and unacceptable behaviors for the client and in developing time-outs (either a set amount of time or until behavior is under control) to reinforce these limits.

19. Help the parents to develop and implement a behavior modification contract with the client in which appropriate behaviors would be rewarded with money or special privileges (e.g., attend an event, go on a family outing) and inappropriate behaviors would

result in fines (e.g., loss of money or privileges).

20. Monitor the parents' follow-through on administering the behavior modification contract and/or time-outs. Give feedback, support, and praise as appropriate.

21. Conduct family sessions during which the family system and its interactions are analyzed. Develop and implement a strategic, structural, or experiential intervention.

22. Monitor the intervention and make adjustments as necessary to ensure its success.

__. _____
   _____

__. _____
   _____

__. _____
   _____

DIAGNOSTIC SUGGESTIONS

Axis I:

313.81	Oppositional Defiant Disorder
312.81	Conduct Disorder/Childhood-Onset Type
312.82	Conduct Disorder/Adolescent-Onset Type
312.9	Disruptive Behavior Disorder NOS
314.01	Attention-Deficit/Hyperactivity Disorder, Predominantly Impulsive Type
314.9	Attention-Deficit/Hyperactivity Disorder NOS
V62.81	Relational Problem NOS
_____	_____
_____	_____

Axis II:

799.9	Diagnosis Deferred
V71.09	No Diagnosis
_____	_____
_____	_____

PEER/SIBLING CONFLICT

BEHAVIORAL DEFINITIONS

1. Frequent, overt, intense fighting (verbal and/or physical) with peers and/or siblings.
2. Peer and/or sibling relationships characterized by fighting, bullying, defiance, revenge, taunting, and incessant teasing.
3. Virtually no friends and those few exhibit similar socially disapproved behavior.
4. General pattern of behavior that is impulsive, intimidating, and unmalleable.
5. Aggressive behavior toward peers that lacks a discernible empathy for others.
6. Failure to respond to praise and encouragement like his/her peers.
7. Argumentative and physically and verbally aggressive attitude toward peers and/or siblings while parents are hostile toward the client, demonstrating a familial pattern of rejection, quarreling, and lack of respect and affection.

—. _____
  _____
  _____
—. _____
  _____
  _____
—. _____
  _____

LONG-TERM GOALS

1. Attain the ability to compete, cooperate, and resolve conflict appropriately with peers and siblings.

2. Develop healthy mechanisms for handling anxiety, tension, frustration, and anger.
3. Obtain the skills required to build positive peer relationships.
4. Bring aggressive behaviors within socially acceptable limits.
5. Form respectful, trusting peer and sibling relationships.

—. _____
   _____
   _____
—. _____
   _____
   _____
—. _____
   _____
   _____

SHORT-TERM OBJECTIVES

1. Develop a working relationship with the therapist in which the client shares thoughts and feelings openly. (1, 4, 11)
2. Decrease the frequency and intensity of aggressive actions toward peers. (1, 2, 3, 4)
3. Identify orally and in writing how he/she would like to be treated by others. (4, 6, 7, 8)
4. Recognize and verbalize the feelings of others as well as his/her own. (4, 7, 8, 11)
5. Increase the frequency of socially appropriate behavior with peers and siblings. (3, 5, 6, 8)

THERAPEUTIC INTERVENTIONS

1. Actively build the level of trust with the client in individual sessions through consistent eye contact, active listening, unconditional positive regard, and warm acceptance to help increase his/her ability to identify and express feelings.
2. Instruct the parents and teachers as the prime reinforcers in the social learning techniques of ignoring the client's aggressive acts except when there is danger of physical injury while making a concerted effort to attend to and praise all nonaggressive, cooperative, and peaceful behavior.
3. Use Anger Control (Berg)* or a similar game to expand

_____

* Berthold Berg, Anger Control Game, Cognitive Counseling Resources, Dayton, Ohio, 1988.

6. Smile, express gratitude, and/or increase the frequency of target behavior when praised and encouraged. (6, 8, 9, 10)

7. Increase the quantity of time spent with peers and siblings without aggressive actions. (2, 5, 8, 12)

8. Verbalize an understanding of the pain that underlies the anger. (10, 11, 12, 13)

9. Decrease the frequency of quarreling and messages of rejection within the family. (15, 16, 17)

10. Increase the parents' verbal and physical demonstrations of affection to the client. (15, 16, 17, 18)

11. The parents develop and implement a behavior modification plan designed to increase the frequency of cooperative social behaviors. (16, 18, 21)

12. Express in family therapy a desire and plan to cooperate with conflict resolution with peers and siblings. (16, 17, 19)

13. The parents terminate alliances with their children that foster sibling conflict. (16, 18, 20)

ways to control the client's aggressive feelings.

4. Educate the client about feelings, focusing on how others feel when they are the focus of aggressive actions.

5. Direct the parents to involve the client in cooperative activities such as sports or scouts.

6. Refer the client to an alternative summer camp that focuses on self-esteem and cooperation with peers.

7. Use therapeutic stories (e.g., Gardner's *Fairy Tales for Today's Children*)* to increase the client's awareness of feelings and ways to cooperate with others.

8. Refer the client to a peer therapy group whose objectives are to increase social sensitivity and behavioral flexibility through group exercises such as strength bombardment, the trust walk, and expressing negative feelings.

9. Assist the client in becoming open and responsive to praise and encouragement.

10. Involve the client in play therapy around themes of cooperation, respect for others, responding to praise, and expression of negative feelings.

---

* R. Gardner, *Fairy Tales for Today's Children* (Cresskill, New Jersey: Creative Therapeutics, 1978).

14. Complete the recommended psychiatric, psychological, or educational testing/evaluation. (22, 23, 24)

15. Comply with the recommendations of the evaluations. (22, 23, 24)

—. _____
_____

—. _____
_____

—. _____
_____

11. Use the Talking, Feeling Doing* game to increase the client's awareness of him/herself and others.

12. Probe the causes for anger in the client's rejection experiences with family and friends.

13. Utilize play therapy techniques to explore the sources of hurt or fear that fuel the client's anger and aggressiveness.

14. Arrange for the client to participate in a behavioral contracting group where contracts for positive peer interaction are developed and reviewed each week. Positive reinforcers are verbal feedback and small concrete rewards.

15. Work with the client's parents in family sessions to eliminate parental messages of rejection and to reduce the quarreling within the family.

16. Refer the client's parents to a parenting class.

17. Assist the parents in verbalizing affection and appropriate praise to the client in family sessions.

18. Conduct weekly contract sessions with the client and his/her parents in which the past week's contract is reviewed and revised for the following week. Give

* Creative Therapeutics, Cresskill, New Jersey, 1973.

feedback and model praise and positive encouragement when appropriate.

19. Facilitate the respectful expression of feelings in a family session that leads to cooperation and peaceful resolution of conflict.

20. Hold family therapy sessions to assess the dynamics and alliances that may underlie peer or sibling conflict.

21. Assist the parents in developing and implementing a behavior modification plan in which the client's positive interaction with peers and siblings is reinforced immediately with tokens to be exchanged for preestablished primary rewards. Monitor and give feedback as indicated.

22. Arrange for a psychiatric, psychological, or educational assessment.

23. Monitor and assist the client and his/her family in following through with the recommendations of the assessment.

__. _____
   _____

__. _____
   _____

__. _____
   _____

DIAGNOSTIC SUGGESTIONS

Axis I:	313.81	Oppositional Defiant Disorder
	312.81	Conduct Disorder/Childhood-Onset Type
	312.82	Conduct Disorder/Adolescent-Onset Type
	312.9	Disruptive Behavior Disorder NOS
	314.01	Attention-Deficit/Hyperactive Disorder, Predominantly Impulsive Type
	314.9	Attention-Deficit/Hyperactivity Disorder NOS
	V62.81	Relational Problem NOS
	V71.02	Child or Adolescent Antisocial Behavior
	315.00	Reading Disorder
	315.9	Learning Disorder NOS
	_____	_____
	_____	_____
Axis II:	799.9	Diagnosis Deferred
	V71.09	No Diagnosis
	_____	_____
	_____	_____

PHOBIA-PANIC/AGORAPHOBIA

BEHAVIORAL DEFINITIONS

1. Fear of being in a place or situation from which escape may be difficult or symptom development (dizziness, depersonalization or derealization, nausea, diarrhea, sweating, heart palpitation, or weakness) may be incapacitating or embarrassing.
2. Resistance to being away from home (especially alone).
3. Avoidance of crowds of people (restaurants, shopping malls, church, theater, and so on).
4. Avoidance of enclosed environments for travel (bus, train, plane, car, and so on).
5. Persistent and unreasonable fear of a specific object or situation because an encounter with the phobic stimulus provokes an immediate anxiety response.
6. Avoidance or endurance of the phobic stimulus with intense anxiety resulting in interference of normal routines or marked distress.

—. _____
   _____
—. _____
   _____
—. _____
   _____

LONG-TERM GOALS

1. Reduce the fear such that the client can independently and freely leave home and comfortably be in public environments with people present.

2. Enable the client to travel away from home in some form of enclosed transportation.
3. Reduce the fear of the specific stimulus object or situation that previously provoked immediate anxiety.
4. Eliminate the interference from normal routines and remove the distress over the feared object or situation.

—. _____
   _____

—. _____
   _____

—. _____
   _____

SHORT-TERM OBJECTIVES

1. Verbalize the fear and focus on describing the specific stimulus for it. (1, 9, 10)

2. Construct a hierarchy of situations that evoke increasing anxiety. (2)

3. Become proficient in progressive deep-muscle relaxation. (3, 4)

4. Identify a nonthreatening, pleasant scene that can be utilized to promote relaxation using guided imagery. (5)

5. Cooperate with systematic desensitization to the anxiety-provoking stimulus object or situation. (5, 6)

6. Engage in in vivo desensitization to the stimulus object or situation. (7)

THERAPEUTIC INTERVENTIONS

1. Discuss and assess the client's fear, its depth, and the stimulus for it.

2. Direct and assist the client in the construction of a hierarchy of anxiety-producing situations.

3. Train the client in progressive relaxation methods.

4. Utilize biofeedback techniques to facilitate the client's relaxation skills.

5. Train the client in guided imagery for anxiety relief.

6. Direct systematic desensitization procedures to reduce the client's phobic response.

7. Assign and/or accompany the client in in vivo desensitization contact with the phobic stimulus object or situation.

7. Leave home without over-whelming anxiety. (6, 7, 8, 20)

8. Encounter the phobic stim-ulus object or situation feel-ing in control, calm, and comfortable. (7, 8)

9. Write out a real or imagined story that describes an encounter with the feared object or situation. (9)

10. Collect pleasant pictures or stories regarding the phobic stimulus and share them in therapy sessions. (11)

11. Enact the feared behavior or encounter the feared sit-uation and freely experi-ence the nondevastating anxiety. (7, 10, 12)

12. Increase the family's sup-port for the client as he/she tolerates more exposure to the phobic stimulus. (13, 14, 15)

13. Identify the symbolic signif-icance the phobic stimulus may have as a basis for fear. (1, 16)

14. Verbalize the separate reali-ties of the irrationally feared object or situation and the emotionally painful experience from the past that is evoked by the phobic stimulus. (1, 17, 18, 19)

8. Review and verbally rein-force the client's progress toward overcoming the anxiety.

9. Use a narrative approach (Michael White)* in which the client writes out the story of his/her fear and then acts out the story with the therapist to externalize the issue. Then assist the client in writing an effective coping resolution to the story that can also be acted out.

10. Play an enjoyable game with the client in the pres-ence of the feared object or situation as a way of desen-sitizing him/her. (This may mean leaving the office to conduct a session.)

11. Structure sessions with the client around using pleas-ant pictures, readings, or storytelling about the feared object or situation as a means of desensitizing him/her to the fear-producing stimulus.

12. Use a strategic intervention (Fisch, Watzlawick, and Weakland)† in which enact-ment of a symptom is pre-scribed, allowing the client to make an obvious display of the anxiety (e.g., if the

---

* D. Epston and M. White, *Narrative Means to Therapeutic Ends* (New York: Norton, 1990).
† R. Fisch, P. Watzlawick, and J. Weakland, *Change* (New York: Norton, 1974).

15. Share the feelings associated with a past emotionally painful situation that is connected to the phobia. (16, 17, 18, 19)

16. Differentiate real from distorted, imagined situations that can produce rational and irrational fear. (17, 18, 19)

17. Verbalize the cognitive beliefs and messages that mediate the anxiety response. (20, 21, 22)

18. Develop positive, healthy, and rational self-talk that reduces fear and allows a behavioral encounter with the avoided stimulus. (21, 22)

19. Responsibly take prescribed psychotropic medication to alleviate the phobic anxiety. (23, 24)

—. _____
   _____

—. _____
   _____

—. _____
   _____

symptom is fear of screaming in a public place, direct the client to go there and do so). Process the client's catastrophizing expectations.

13. Hold family sessions in which the family is instructed to give support as the client faces the phobic stimulus and not to give support if the client panics and fails to face the fear (Pitman).* Offer encouragement, support, and redirection as required.

14. Assist the family in overcoming the tendency to reinforce the client's phobia and as the phobia decreases, instruct them in constructive ways to reward the client's progress.

15. Assess and confront family members for instances when they model phobic fear responses for the client in the presence of the feared object or situation.

16. Probe, discuss, and interpret the possible symbolic meaning of the phobic stimulus object or situation.

17. Clarify and differentiate between the client's current irrational fear and past emotional pain.

_____

* F. Pittman, *Turning Points* (New York: Norton, 1987), pp. 237–245.

18. Encourage the client to share feelings from the past through active listening, positive regard, and questioning.

19. Reinforce the client's insights into past emotional pain and present anxiety.

20. Train the client in coping strategies (diversion, deep breathing, positive self-talk, muscle relaxation, and so on).

21. Identify the distorted schemas and related automatic thoughts that mediate the client's anxiety response.

22. Train the client in revising core schemas using cognitive restructuring techniques.

23. Arrange for the prescription of psychotropic medications for the client.

24. Monitor the client for medication compliance and effectiveness.

___. _____

_____

___. _____

_____

___. _____

_____

DIAGNOSTIC SUGGESTIONS

Axis I:	300.22	Panic Without Agoraphobia
	300.21	Panic With Agoraphobia
	300.29	Simple Phobia
	_____	_____
	_____	_____

Axis II:	799.9	Diagnosis Deferred
	V71.09	No Diagnosis
	_____	_____
	_____	_____

PHYSICAL ABUSE VICTIM

BEHAVIORAL DEFINITIONS

1. Confirmed self-report or account by others of assault (e.g., hitting, burning, kicking, slapping, or torture) by an older person.
2. Bruises or wounds as evidence of victimization.
3. Self-reports of being injured by a supposed caregiver coupled with feelings of fear and social withdrawal.
4. Significant increase in the frequency and severity of aggressive behaviors toward peers or adults.
5. Recurrent and intrusive distressing recollections of the abuse.
6. Feelings of anger, rage, or fear when in contact with the perpetrator.
7. Pronounced disturbance of mood and affect (i.e., frequent and prolonged periods of depression, irritability, anxiety, and apathetic withdrawal).
8. Appearance of regressive behaviors (e.g., thumb sucking, baby talk, bed-wetting).
9. Sleep disturbances (e.g., difficulty falling asleep, refusal to sleep alone, night terrors, recurrent distressing nightmares).
10. Running away to avoid further physical assaults.

—. _____
   _____

—. _____
   _____

—. _____
   _____

LONG-TERM GOALS

1. Terminate the physical abuse.
2. Rebuild the client's sense of self-worth and remove the overwhelming sense of fear, shame, and sadness.
3. Resolve the client's feelings of fear and depression while improving communication and the boundaries of respect within the family.
4. Remove the client from the environment where the abuse is occurring and provide him/her with a safe haven.
5. Establish limits on the punishment of the client such that no physical harm can occur and respect for his/her rights is maintained.
6. Eliminate denial in the client and his/her family, putting the responsibility for the abuse on the perpetrator and allowing the victim to feel supported.
7. Reduce the client's displays of aggression which reflect his/her abuse and keep others at an emotional distance.
8. Build self-esteem and a sense of empowerment in the client as manifested by an increased number of positive self-descriptive statements and greater participation in extracurricular activities.

—. _____
   _____
—. _____
   _____
—. _____
   _____

SHORT-TERM OBJECTIVES

1. Tell the entire account of the abuse. (1, 2, 3, 4, 5)
2. Identify the nature, frequency, and duration of the abuse. (3, 4, 5, 6, 7)
3. Identify and express the feelings connected to the abuse. (1, 2, 3, 10, 22)
4. Stabilize the client's mood and decrease the emotional

THERAPEUTIC INTERVENTIONS

1. Actively build the level of trust with the client in individual sessions through consistent eye contact, active listening, unconditional positive regard, and warm acceptance to help increase his/her ability to identify and express feelings.
2. Explore, encourage, and support the client in ver-

intensity connected to the abuse. (1, 2, 3, 17, 18)

5. Verbalize the way physical abuse has impacted the client's life. (2, 3, 10, 22)

6. Terminate the client's verbalizations of excuses for the perpetrator. (8, 9)

7. The parents verbalize the establishment of appropriate disciplinary boundaries to ensure protection of the client. (7, 11, 12)

8. Decrease the client's feelings of shame and guilt by affirming the perpetrator as responsible for the abuse. (2, 8, 9, 11, 12)

9. Have the perpetrator take responsibility for the abuse. (8, 13, 15, 16, 17)

10. Have the perpetrator ask for forgiveness and pledge respect for disciplinary boundaries. (9, 12, 16, 17)

11. Have the perpetrator agree to seek treatment. (8, 14, 15, 24, 25)

12. Express forgiveness of the perpetrator and others connected with the abuse while insisting on respect for the client's own right to safety in the future. (16, 17, 18, 19, 21)

13. Reduce the rage and aggressiveness that stems from feelings of helplessness related to physical abuse. (16, 25, 27)

bally expressing and clarifying his/her feelings associated with the abuse.

3. Utilize individual play therapy sessions to provide the client with the opportunity to express and work through feelings of hurt, fear, and anger related to the abuse.

4. Report physical abuse to the appropriate child protection agency, criminal justice officials, or medical professionals.

5. Consult with the family, a physician, criminal justice officials, or child protection case managers to assess the veracity of the physical abuse charges.

6. Assess whether the perpetrator should be removed from the client's home.

7. Implement the necessary steps (e.g., removal of the client from the home) to protect the client and other children in the home from future physical abuse.

8. Actively confront and challenge denial within the family system.

9. Confront the client about making excuses for the perpetrator's abuse and accepting blame for it.

10. Assess the client's need for psychotropic medication and, if necessary, arrange for a prescription.

14. Verbalize an understanding of how poor anger control continues the cycle of violence and distrust present in the extended family. (27, 31)

15. Reduce the depressive behaviors of flat affect, poor concentration, low energy, and social withdrawal. (20, 21, 23, 26)

16. Increase the self-esteem as evidenced by more frequent positive self-descriptive statements, improved eye contact, and a stronger voice. (20, 23, 24, 25)

17. Increase the self-confidence as shown by more active socialization, faster decision making, and a verbalized positive outlook on the future. (22, 24, 25, 26, 30)

18. Decrease the statements of being a victim while increasing the statements that reflect personal empowerment. (11, 21, 22, 24)

19. Verbalize an understanding of the loss of trust in all relationships that results from abuse by a parent. (2, 3, 18, 27, 28)

20. Increase the level of trust of others as shown by increased socialization and a greater number of friendships. (18, 25, 27, 28, 30)

21. Increase contacts outside the family and build social networks. (26, 28, 30)

11. Empower the client by reinforcing the steps to take to protect him/herself.

12. Counsel the client's family member(s) about appropriate disciplinary boundaries.

13. Assess the family dynamics and identify the stress factors or precipitating events that contributed to the emergence of the abuse.

14. Require the perpetrator to participate in a child abuser's group.

15. Evaluate the possibility of substance abuse problems within the family.

16. Hold a family therapy session where the client and/or therapist confront the perpetrator with the abuse.

17. Hold a family session where the perpetrator apologizes to the client and/or other family member(s) for the abuse.

18. Assign the client to write a letter expressing feelings of hurt, fear, and anger to the perpetrator and process it with the therapist.

19. Assign the client to write a forgiveness letter and/or complete a forgiveness exercise in which he/she verbalizes forgiveness to the perpetrator and/or significant family member(s) while asserting the right to safety. Process this with the therapist.

20. Elicit and reinforce support and nurturance for the client from other key family member(s).

___. _____
      _____
___. _____
      _____
___. _____
      _____

21. Assign the client a letting-go exercise in which a symbol of the abuse is disposed of or destroyed. Process this with the therapist.

22. Refer the client to a victim support group with other children to assist them in realizing that they are not alone in their experience.

23. Assist the client in identifying a basis for self-worth by reviewing his/her talents, importance to others, and intrinsic spiritual value.

24. Reinforce positive statements the client has made about him/herself and the future.

25. Reinforce the client's self-worth by relating to him/her with unconditional positive regard, genuine warmth, and active listening.

26. Encourage the client in making plans for the future that involve interacting with his/her peers and family.

27. Assist the client in making discriminating judgments that allow for the trust of some people rather than distrust of all.

28. Teach the client the share-check method of building trust, in which a degree of shared information is related to a proven level of trustworthiness.

29. Arrange for psychological testing with the client and/or family member(s) to rule out the presence of severe psychological disorders.

30. Encourage the client to participate in positive peer groups or extracurricular activities.

31. Construct a multigenerational family genogram that identifies physical abuse within the extended family to help the client realize that he/she is not the only victim and to help the perpetrator recognize the cycle of violence.

__. _____
    _____

__. _____
    _____

__. _____
    _____

DIAGNOSTIC SUGGESTIONS

Axis I:	309.81	Posttraumatic Stress Disorder
	308.3	Acute Stress Disorder
	300.4	Dysthymic Disorder
	296.xx	Major Depressive Disorder
	311	Depressive Disorder NOS
	300.02	Generalized Anxiety Disorder
	V61.21	Physical Abuse of Child, 995.5 Victim
	307.47	Nightmare Disorder
	313.81	Oppositional Defiant Disorder
	312.81	Conduct Disorder/Childhood-Onset Type
	312.82	Conduct Disorder/Adolescent-Onset Type
	300.6	Depersonalization Disorder
	300.15	Dissociative Disorder NOS
	_____	_____
	_____	_____
Axis II:	799.9	Diagnosis Deferred
	V71.09	No Diagnosis
	_____	_____
	_____	_____

PSYCHOTICISM

BEHAVIORAL DEFINITIONS

1. Bizarre thought content (delusions of grandeur, persecution, reference, influence, control, somatic sensations, or infidelity).
2. Illogical form of thought or speech (loose association of ideas in speech; incoherence; illogical thinking; vague, abstract, or repetitive speech; neologisms; perseverations; clanging).
3. Perception disturbance (hallucinations, primarily auditory but occasionally visual or olfactory).
4. Disturbed affect (blunted, none, flattened, or inappropriate).
5. Lost sense of self (loss of ego boundaries, lack of identity, blatant confusion).
6. Diminished volition (inadequate interest, drive, or ability to follow a course of action to its logical conclusion; pronounced ambivalence or cessation of goal-directed activity).
7. Relationship withdrawal (withdrawal from involvement with the external world and preoccupation with egocentric ideas and fantasies; alienation feelings).
8. Poor social skills (misinterpretation of the actions or motives of others; maintaining emotional distance from others; feeling awkward and threatened in most social situations and embarrassment of others by the client's failure to recognize the impact of his/her behavior).
9. Inadequate control over sexual, aggressive, or frightening thoughts, feelings, or impulses (blatantly sexual or aggressive fantasies; fears of impending doom; acting out sexual or aggressive impulses in an unpredictable and unusual manner, often directed toward family and friends).
10. Psychomotor abnormalities (a marked decrease in reactivity to the environment; various catatonic patterns such as stupor, rigidity, excitement, posturing, or negativism; unusual mannerisms or grimacing).

—. _____
  _____
—. _____
  _____
—. _____
  _____

LONG-TERM GOALS

1. Control or eliminate active psychotic symptoms such that supervised functioning is positive and medication is taken consistently.
2. Significantly reduce or eliminate hallucinations and/or delusions.
3. Eliminate acute, reactive psychotic symptoms and return to normal functioning in affect, thinking, and relating.
4. Interact appropriately in social situations and improve the realistic understanding of and reaction to the behaviors and motives of others.
5. Attain control over disturbing thoughts, feelings, and impulses.

—. _____
  _____
—. _____
  _____
—. _____
  _____

SHORT-TERM OBJECTIVES

1. Accept and understand that the distressing symptoms are due to mental illness. (1, 2, 3, 8)
2. Understand the necessity for taking antipsychotic medications and agree to cooperate with prescribed care. (1, 4, 5, 6)

THERAPEUTIC INTERVENTIONS

1. Assess the pervasiveness of the client's thought disorder through a clinical interview and/or arrange for psychological testing.
2. Determine if the client's psychosis is of a brief reactive nature or long term with prodromal and reactive elements.

3. Take antipsychotic medications consistently. (4, 5, 6)

4. Begin to show limited social functioning by responding appropriately to friendly encounters. (4, 7, 8, 22, 29)

5. Gradually return to a premorbid level of functioning and participate in age-appropriate social and academic activities. (7, 9, 16, 17, 29)

6. Increase the family's positive support of the client to reduce the chances of acute exacerbation of the psychotic episode. (10, 11, 18, 28)

7. Increase the frequency of the parents communicating to the client with direct eye contact, clear language, and complete thoughts. (12, 15)

8. Decrease the parents' contradictory messages to the client and increase the verbal and nonverbal consistency of communication. (10, 12, 15, 18)

9. Terminate hostile, critical responses from the parents to the client and increase the statements of praise, optimism, and affirmation. (13, 14, 28)

10. Stay current with schoolwork, completing assignments and interacting appropriately with peers and teachers. (16, 17, 24)

11. Increase support in the school setting, with teachers being more understand-

3. Explore the client's family history for serious mental illness.

4. Arrange for an appropriate level of residential care for the client, if necessary.

5. Arrange for the administration of appropriate psychotropic medications.

6. Monitor the client for medication compliance and redirect if he/she is non-compliant.

7. Monitor the client's daily level of functioning (i.e., reality orientation, personal hygiene, social interactions, affect appropriateness) and give feedback that either redirects or reinforces the behavior.

8. Provide supportive therapy characterized by genuine warmth, understanding, and acceptance to reduce the client's distrust, alleviate fears, and promote openness.

9. Use role play and behavioral rehearsal of social situations to explore and teach the client alternative positive social interactions with family and friends.

10. Arrange for family therapy sessions to educate them regarding the client's illness, treatment, and prognosis.

11. Encourage family members to share their feelings of frustration, guilt, fear, or depression surrounding the client's mental illness and behavior patterns.

ing of the client's illness and verbalizing acceptance of him/her. (16, 17)

12. Verbally identify the stressors that contributed to the reactive psychosis. (8, 18, 19, 20, 29, 30)

13. Verbalize reduced anxiety over and increased confidence in the ability to cope with environmental stressors. (18, 19, 20, 27, 29)

14. Think more clearly as demonstrated by logical, coherent speech. (5, 22, 24, 25, 27)

15. Report a diminishing or absence of hallucinations and/or delusions. (5, 20, 21, 24)

16. Verbalize an understanding of the underlying needs, conflicts, and emotions that support the irrational beliefs. (19, 21, 23, 27, 30)

17. Demonstrate control over inappropriate thoughts, feelings, and impulses by verbalizing a reduced frequency of occurrence. (14, 21, 26)

___. _____
_____

___. _____
_____

___. _____
_____

12. Assist the family in avoiding double-bind messages that are inconsistent and contradictory, resulting in increased anxiety, confusion, and psychotic symptoms in the client.

13. Hold family therapy sessions to reduce the atmosphere of criticism and hostility toward the client and promote an understanding of the client and his/her illness.

14. Support the parents in setting firm limits without hostility on the client's inappropriate aggressive or sexual behavior.

15. Confront the parents in family therapy when their communication is indirect and disjointed, leaving the client confused and anxious.

16. Arrange for and/or encourage ongoing academic training while the client is receiving psychological treatment.

17. Contact school personnel (having obtained the necessary confidentiality releases) to educate them regarding the client's unusual behavior and his/her need for an accepting, supportive environment.

18. Assist the client in identifying threats in the environment and develop a plan with the family to reduce these stressors.

19. Probe the causes for the client's reactive psychosis.

20. Explore the client's feelings about the stressors that triggered the psychotic episodes.

21. Assist in restructuring the client's irrational beliefs by reviewing reality-based evidence and misinterpretation.

22. Differentiate for the client between the sources of stimuli from self-generated messages and the reality of the external world.

23. Probe the client's underlying needs and feelings (e.g., inadequacy, rejection, anxiety, guilt).

24. Encourage the client to focus on the reality of the external world as opposed to distorted fantasy.

25. Gently confront the client's illogical thoughts and speech to refocus disordered thinking.

26. Set firm limits on the client's inappropriate aggressive or sexual behavior that emanates from a lack of impulse control or a misperception of reality.

27. Interpret the client's inaccurate perceptions or bizarre associations as reflective of unspoken fears of rejection or losing control.

28. Encourage the parents to involve the client in here-and-now-based social and recreational activities (e.g.,

intramural sports, after-school enrichment programs, YMCA structured programs).

29. Utilize individual play therapy sessions to provide the client with the opportunity to work through, clarify, and express his/her feelings.

30. Explore the client's history for significant separations, losses, or traumas.

__. _____

_____

__. _____

_____

__. _____

_____

DIAGNOSTIC SUGGESTIONS

Axis I:	297.1	Delusional Disorder
	298.8	Brief Psychotic Disorder
	295.xx	Schizophrenia
	295.30	Schizophrenia, Paranoid Type
	295.70	Schizoaffective Disorder
	295.40	Schizophreniform Disorder
	296.xx	Bipolar I Disorder
	296.89	Bipolar II Disorder
	296.24	Major Depressive Disorder, Single Episode With Psychotic Features
	296.34	Major Depressive Disorder, Recurrent With Psychotic Features
	310.1	Personality Change Due to (Axis III Disorder)
	_____	_____
	_____	_____
Axis II:	799.9	Diagnosis Deferred
	V71.09	No Diagnosis
	_____	_____
	_____	_____

RUNAWAY

BEHAVIORAL DEFINITIONS

1. Running away from home for a day or more without parental permission.
2. Pattern of running to the noncustodial parent, relative, or friend when conflicts arise with the custodial parent or guardian.
3. Running away from home and crossing state lines.
4. Running away from home overnight at least twice while living in parents' or guardian's home (or once without returning for a lengthy period).

—. _____

_____

—. _____

_____

—. _____

_____

LONG-TERM GOALS

1. Develop a closer, more caring relationship between the parents and client.
2. Reduce the level, frequency, and degree of family conflicts.
3. Attain the necessary skills to cope with family stress without resorting to the flight response.
4. Terminate any abuse of the client and establish a nurturing family environment with appropriate boundaries.
5. Eliminate the runaway behavior.
6. Begin the process of healthy separation from the family.

—. _____
  _____
  _____

—. _____
  _____
  _____

—. _____
  _____
  _____

SHORT-TERM OBJECTIVES

1. Develop sufficient trust in the therapist to verbalize the pain causing the need to escape from the home environment. (1, 2, 10)

2. Decrease impulsive reactions to conflictual situations. (1, 2, 3, 4)

3. Increase communications and the level of understanding between the client and his/her parents. (2, 4, 5, 7)

4. The client and his/her parents verbalize responsibility for their individual contributions to the conflicts between them. (5, 7, 9)

5. Terminate any physical and/or sexual abuse of the client. (5, 6, 7, 9)

6. Identify the client's unmet needs within the family. (1, 2, 10, 11)

7. Decrease the parents' messages of rejection toward the client. (9, 12, 13, 14)

THERAPEUTIC INTERVENTIONS

1. Actively build the level of trust with the client in individual sessions through consistent eye contact, active listening, unconditional positive regard, and warm acceptance to help increase his/her ability to identify and express feelings.

2. Probe causes for the client's pain that prompt the runaway behavior.

3. Train the client in alternative ways to handle conflictual situations and assist in implementing them in his/her daily life.

4. Ask the client to list all possible ways of handling conflictual situations and process this list with the therapist.

5. Probe the client and his/her family for any occurrence of physical or sexual abuse to the client.

6. Arrange for the client to be placed in respite care or another secure setting, if

8. Increase the frequency of statements that affirm a sense of personal value. (11, 12, 15, 16)

9. The parents identify ways they can make the client feel valued and cherished within the family. (12, 13, 14, 15)

10. Verbalize a plan to become more responsible and mature in behavior. (11, 16, 17, 18)

11. Verbalize angry feelings connected to the family and how it functions. (1, 2, 20, 21)

12. Identify specifically how runaway behavior rescues the parents from focusing on themselves. (22, 23, 24)

13. Verbally agree to and then implement the structural or strategic recommendations of the therapist for the family. (24, 25)

14. Cooperate with the evaluations for substance abuse, ADHD, or psychosis. (7, 26, 27)

15. Comply with all the recommendations resulting from the evaluations. (6, 13, 26, 27)

___. _____
   _____

___. _____
   _____

___. _____
   _____

necessary, while the family works in family therapy to resolve conflicts.

7. Evaluate the parents for chemical dependence and its effect on the client.

8. Assign the client to attend a problem-solving psychoeducational group.

9. Assist the client and his/her parents in accepting responsibility for their individual contributions to the conflicts between them.

10. Ask the client to make a list of his/her needs in the family that are not met. Process the list in an individual session and at an appropriate later time in a family session.

11. Encourage the client to begin meeting those unmet needs that would be age appropriate for him/her to meet.

12. Conduct family therapy sessions with the client and his/her parents to facilitate healthy, positive communications.

13. Ask the client's parents to attend a parenting class.

14. Assign the client's parents to read books on parenting (*P.E.T.* by Gordon or *Raising Self-Reliant Children in a Self-Indulgent World* by Glenn and Nelsen) and process what they have learned.

15. Conduct sessions with the parents to assist them in developing ways to make the client feel more valued as an individual and as part of the family.

16. Help the client develop and implement specific constructive ways to interact with his/her parents.

17. Confront the client when he/she is not taking responsibility for him/herself in family conflicts.

18. Probe the client's fears about becoming more independent and responsible for him/herself.

19. Work with the parents to help them find ways to assist in the advancement of the client's maturity and independence.

20. Support and encourage the client when he/she begins to appropriately verbalize angry or other negative feelings.

21. Educate the client in how to identify his/her feelings and the value of expressing them in appropriate ways.

22. Assist the client to become more aware of his/her role in the family and how it takes the focus off the parents.

23. Facilitate family therapy sessions with the objective of revealing underlying conflicts to release the client from being the symptom bearer.

24. Conduct family therapy sessions in which a structural intervention is developed, assigned, and then implemented by the client's family. The therapist will monitor and adjust the intervention as required.

25. Develop a strategic intervention and have the client's family implement it. The therapist will monitor and adjust the intervention as needed.

26. Arrange for an evaluation of the client for substance abuse, ADHD, affective disorder, or psychotic process.

27. Monitor the client's and family's compliance with the recommendations resulting from the evaluations.

___. _____

_____

___. _____

_____

___. _____

_____

DIAGNOSTIC SUGGESTIONS

Axis I:	314.01	Attention-Deficit/Hyperactivity Disorder, Predominantly Hyperactive-Impulsive Type
	312.81	Conduct Disorder/Childhood-Onset Type
	312.82	Conduct Disorder/Adolescent-Onset Type
	313.81	Oppositional Defiant Disorder
	300.4	Dysthymic Disorder
	309.24	Adjustment Disorder With Anxiety
	309.4	Adjustment Disorder With Mixed Disturbance of Emotions and Conduct
	312.30	Impulse-Control Disorder NOS
	V61.20	Parent-Child Relational Problem
	V61.21	Physical Abuse of Child, 995.54 Victim
	V61.21	Sexual Abuse of Child, 995.53 Victim
	V61.21	Neglect of Child, 995.52 Victim
	_____	_____
	_____	_____
Axis II:	301.83	Borderline Personality Disorder
	799.9	Diagnosis Deferred
	V71.09	No Diagnosis
	_____	_____
	_____	_____

SCHOOL REFUSAL

BEHAVIORAL DEFINITIONS

1. Persistent reluctance or refusal to attend school because of a desire to remain at home with the parent(s).
2. Marked emotional distress and repeated complaints (e.g., crying, regressive behaviors, temper outbursts, pleading with parent(s) not to go to school) when anticipating separation from home to attend school or after arrival at school.
3. Frequent somatic complaints (e.g., headaches, stomachaches, nausea) associated with attending school or in anticipation of school attendance.
4. Excessive clinging or shadowing of parent(s) when anticipating leaving home or after arriving at school.
5. Frequent negative comments about school and/or repeated questioning of the necessity of going to school.
6. Persistent and unrealistic expression of fear that a future calamity will separate the client from his/her parent(s) if the client attends school (e.g., the client or his/her parent(s) will be lost, kidnapped, killed, or the victim of an accident).
7. Low self-esteem and lack of self-confidence that contribute to the fear of attending school and being separated from the parent(s).
8. Verbalization of a fear of failure and anxiety regarding academic achievement accompanying the refusal to attend school.

—. _____
   _____
—. _____
   _____
—. _____
   _____

LONG-TERM GOALS

1. Attend school on a consistent, full-time basis.
2. Eliminate anxiety and the expression of fears prior to leaving home and after arriving at school.
3. Cease the temper outbursts, regressive behaviors, complaints, and pleading associated with attending school.
4. Eliminate the somatic complaints associated with attending school.
5. Resolve the core conflicts or traumas contributing to the emergence of the school refusal.
6. Verbalize positive statements about accomplishments and experiences at school.
7. Engage in independent behaviors (work on school assignments alone, participate in extracurricular activities, play with peers).
8. The parent(s) establish and maintain appropriate parent-child boundaries, setting firm, consistent limits when the client exhibits temper tantrums and passive-aggressive behaviors associated with attending school.

—. _____
   _____
   _____
—. _____
   _____
   _____
—. _____
   _____

SHORT-TERM OBJECTIVES

1. Complete psychological testing and an assessment interview. (1, 3, 4)
2. Complete psychoeducational testing. (2, 3)
3. The parent(s) and school officials effectively implement a systematic desensitization program. (5, 6, 7)
4. Comply with a systematic desensitization program

THERAPEUTIC INTERVENTIONS

1. Arrange for psychological testing of the client to assess the severity of anxiety, depression, or gross psychopathology and gain greater insight into the underlying dynamics contributing to school refusal.
2. Arrange for psychoeducational testing of the client to rule out the presence of learning disabilities.

and begin to attend school for increasingly longer periods of time. (4, 5, 6, 7, 9)

5. The parent(s) and school officials implement a contingency plan to deal with temper tantrums, crying spells, or excessive clinging after arriving at school. (6, 7, 21, 22, 23)

6. Decrease the intensity of the crying spells and temper outbursts associated with attending school. (6, 21, 23)

7. Increase the positive statements about accomplishments and experiences at school. (4, 7, 8, 9)

8. Decrease the frequency of negative comments and questions about attending school. (6, 20, 21)

9. Reduce or eliminate the irrational anxiety or fears. (10, 11, 12, 13, 14)

10. Verbally acknowledge how the fears related to attending school are irrational or unrealistic. (10, 11, 12)

11. The parent(s) and school officials follow through with a contingency plan to manage the client's somatic complaints. (15, 16, 17)

12. Decrease the frequency of verbalized somatic complaints. (15, 16, 17)

13. Understand and verbally recognize the secondary gain that results from somatic complaints. (16, 17, 20)

3. Give feedback to the client and his/her family regarding the results of the psychological testing.

4. Actively build the level of trust with the client in individual sessions through consistent eye contact, active listening, unconditional positive regard, and warm acceptance to help increase his/her ability to identify and express feelings.

5. Design and implement a systematic desensitization program to help the client manage his/her anxiety and gradually attend school for longer periods of time.

6. Consult with the parent(s) and school officials to develop a plan to manage the client's emotional distress and negative outbursts after arriving at school (e.g., the parent ceases lengthy good-byes, the client goes to the principal's office to calm down).

7. Reward the client for attending school for increasingly longer periods of time.

8. Consult with the teacher in the initial stages of treatment about planning an assignment that will provide the client with an increased chance of success.

9. Utilize the teacher's aide or a positive peer role model to provide one-on-one attention for the client and help decrease the fear and anxiety about attending school.

14. The parent(s) reinforce the client's autonomous behaviors and set limits on overly dependent behaviors. (18, 20, 21, 22)

15. The parents cease sending inconsistent messages about school attendance and begin to set firm, consistent limits on excessive clinging, pleading, crying, and temper tantrums. (18, 19, 21, 22, 25)

16. The enmeshed or overly protective parent identifies and verbally recognizes how he/she reinforces overly dependent behaviors. (19, 20, 21)

17. Increase the time spent between the client and the disengaged parent in play, school, or work activities. (18, 19, 23, 24)

18. Verbalize an understanding of how current fears and anxiety about attending school are associated with past separation, loss, or trauma. (4, 26, 27, 30, 31)

19. Identify and express the feelings connected with past unresolved separation, loss, or trauma. (27, 28, 29, 30, 31)

20. Increase the frequency and duration of time spent in independent play or activities away from the parent(s) or home. (21, 32, 33)

21. Increase the participation in school or positive peer group activities. (32, 33)

10. Explore the irrational cognitive messages that produce the client's anxiety or fear.

11. Assist the client in realizing that his/her fears about attending school are irrational or unrealistic.

12. Assist the client in developing reality-based cognitive messages that increase his/her self-confidence to cope with anxiety or fear.

13. Train the client in relaxation techniques or guided imagery to reduce his/her anxiety and fears.

14. Assist the client in developing and implementing positive self-talk as a means of managing the anxiety or fears associated with school refusal.

15. Consult with the parent(s) and school officials to develop a contingency plan to manage the client's somatic complaints (e.g., ignore them, take the client's temperature, redirect the client back to the task, send the client to the nurse's office).

16. Refocus the client's discussion from physical complaints to emotional conflicts and the expression of feelings.

17. Assist the client and his/her parent(s) in developing insight into the secondary gain received from physical illnesses, complaints, and the like.

22. Increase the positive self-descriptive statements. (4, 14, 32)

23. Increase communication, intimacy, and consistency between the parents. (18, 24)

24. Take medication as prescribed by the physician. (34, 35, 36)

—. _____
   _____

—. _____
   _____

—. _____
   _____

18. Conduct family therapy sessions to assess the dynamics contributing to the emergence of the school refusal.

19. Utilize a family-sculpting technique in which the client describes the behavior of each family member in a specific scene of his/her choosing, to assess the family dynamics.

20. Identify how enmeshed or overly protective parent(s) reinforce the client's dependency and irrational fears.

21. Encourage the parent(s) to reinforce the client's autonomous behaviors (e.g., attend school, work alone on school assignments) and set limits on overly dependent behaviors (e.g., the client insisting that the parent enter the classroom).

22. Counsel the parent(s) about setting firm, consistent limits on the client's temper outbursts, manipulative behaviors, or excessive clinging.

23. Give a directive to the disengaged or distant parent to transport the client to school in the morning; contact the parent's employer, if necessary, to gain permission for this.

24. Assess the marital dyad for possible conflict and the triangulation that places the focus on the client's symptoms and away from discord.

25. Use a paradoxical intervention (e.g., instruct the enmeshed parent to spoon-feed the client each morning) to work around the family's resistance and disengage the client from an overly protective parent.

26. Assess whether the client's anxiety and fear about attending school are associated with a previously unresolved separation, loss, trauma, or realistic danger.

27. Explore, encourage, and support the client in verbally expressing and clarifying his/her feelings associated with a past separation, loss, trauma, or realistic danger.

28. Assign the client to write a letter to express his/her feelings about a past separation, loss, trauma, or danger; process it with the therapist.

29. Request that the client perform a letting-go exercise in which a symbol of a past separation, loss, or trauma is destroyed; process this with the therapist.

30. Utilize individual play therapy sessions to provide the client with the opportunity to express and work through his/her feelings and fears.

31. Interpret the feelings and fears expressed in play therapy and relate them to the client's anxiety about attending school.

32. Encourage the client's participation in extracurricular and positive peer group activities.

33. Give the client a directive to spend a specified period of time with his/her peers after school or on weekends.

34. Arrange for psychotropic medication for the client, if necessary.

35. Monitor the client for compliance, side effects, and effectiveness of the medication.

36. Refer the client for a medical examination to rule out genuine health problems.

__. _____
   _____

__. _____
   _____

__. _____
   _____

DIAGNOSTIC SUGGESTIONS

Axis I:	309.21	Separation Anxiety
	300.02	Generalized Anxiety Disorder
	300.23	Social Phobia
	296.xx	Major Depressive Disorder
	300.40	Dysthymic Disorder
	300.82	Somatization Disorder
	300.82	Undifferentiated Somatoform Disorder
	309.81	Posttraumatic Stress Disorder
	_____	_____
	_____	_____
Axis II:	799.9	Diagnosis Deferred
	V71.09	No Diagnosis
	_____	_____
	_____	_____

SEPARATION ANXIETY

BEHAVIORAL DEFINITIONS

1. Excessive emotional distress and repeated complaints (e.g., crying, regressive behaviors, pleading with parents to stay, temper tantrums) when anticipating separation from home or major attachment figures.
2. Persistent and unrealistic worry about possible harm occurring to major attachment figures or excessive fear that they will leave and not return.
3. Persistent and unrealistic fears expressed that a future calamity will separate the client from a major attachment figure (e.g., the client or his/her parent will be lost, kidnapped, killed, or the victim of an accident).
4. Repeated complaints and heightened distress (e.g., pleading to go home, demanding to see or call a parent) after separation from home or the attachment figure has occurred.
5. Persistent fear or avoidance of being alone as manifested by excessive clinging and shadowing of a major attachment figure.
6. Frequent reluctance or refusal to go to sleep without being near a major attachment figure or refusal to sleep away from home.
7. Recurrent nightmares centering around the theme of separation.
8. Frequent somatic complaints (e.g., headaches, stomachaches, nausea) when separation from home or the attachment figure is anticipated.
9. Excessive need for reassurance about safety and protection from possible harm or danger.
10. Low self-esteem and a lack of self-confidence that contributes to the fear of being alone or participating in social activities.
11. Excessive shrinking from unfamiliar or new situations.

___. _____
     _____
     _____
___. _____
     _____
     _____
___. _____
     _____

LONG-TERM GOALS

1. Eliminate the anxiety and expression of fears when a separation is anticipated or occurs.
2. Tolerate separation from attachment figures without exhibiting heightened emotional distress, regressive behaviors, temper outbursts, or pleading.
3. Eliminate the somatic complaints associated with separation.
4. Manage nighttime fears effectively as evidenced by the client remaining calm, sleeping in his/her own bed, and not attempting to go into the attachment figure's room at night.
5. Resolve the core conflicts or traumas contributing to the emergence of the separation anxiety.
6. Participate in extracurricular or peer group activities and spend time in independent play on a regular, consistent basis.
7. The parents establish and maintain appropriate parent-child boundaries and set firm, consistent limits when the client exhibits temper outbursts or manipulative behaviors around separation points.

___. _____
     _____
     _____
___. _____
     _____
     _____
___. _____
     _____

SHORT-TERM OBJECTIVES

1. Complete psychological testing. (1, 2)

2. Develop and implement behavioral and cognitive strategies to reduce or eliminate irrational anxiety or fears. (3, 4, 5, 6, 7)

3. Verbally acknowledge how the fears are irrational or unrealistic. (3, 4, 5, 6, 7)

4. Reduce the frequency and severity of crying, clinging, temper tantrums, and verbalized fears when separated from attachment figures. (3, 4, 6, 8, 32)

5. Decrease the frequency of crying spells and temper outbursts at times of separation. (5, 21, 25)

6. Increase the frequency and duration of time spent in independent play away from major attachment figures. (9, 20)

7. Increase the participation in extracurricular or positive peer group activities away from home. (9, 10, 11, 13)

8. Increase the frequency and duration of contacts with peers away from the presence of the attachment figure. (9, 10, 11, 12)

9. Decrease the frequency of verbalized, somatic complaints. (15, 16, 19, 38)

THERAPEUTIC INTERVENTIONS

1. Arrange for psychological testing to assess the severity of the client's anxiety and gain greater insight into the underlying dynamics contributing to the symptoms.

2. Give feedback to the client and his/her family regarding the results of the psychological testing.

3. Explore the irrational cognitive messages that produce anxiety or fear in the client.

4. Assist the client in developing reality-based cognitive messages that increase his/her self-confidence to cope with the anxiety or fears.

5. Train the client in relaxation techniques or guided imagery to reduce anxiety.

6. Assist the client in developing positive self-talk as a means of managing the anxiety or fears associated with separation.

7. Utilize biofeedback techniques to increase the client's relaxation skills and decrease the level of anxiety and resultant somatic ailments.

8. Assist the client in realizing how his/her fears are irrational or unrealistic.

9. Give the client directives to spend gradually longer peri-

10. Understand and verbally recognize the secondary gain that results from somatic complaints. (15, 16, 38)

11. Increase school attendance as evidenced by a decreased frequency of unexcused absences. (13, 15, 20, 21)

12. Begin to manage nighttime fears more effectively as evidenced by fewer visits to the attachment figure's room at night. (5, 6, 8, 14, 20)

13. The parents reinforce the client's autonomous behavior and set limits on overly dependent behaviors. (13, 17, 20, 21, 25)

14. The enmeshed or overly protective parent(s) identify how they reinforce irrational fears or dependent behaviors. (17, 18, 19, 23, 24)

15. Increase the time spent between the client and the disengaged parent in play, school, or work activities. (22, 23, 25)

16. The parents begin to set limits on the client's excessive clinging, whining, pleading, and temper tantrums. (20, 21, 23, 24, 25)

17. Verbalize how current anxiety and fears are associated with past separation, loss, or trauma. (26, 27, 28, 29, 34)

ods of time in independent play or with friends after school.

10. Encourage the client to participate in extracurricular or peer group activities.

11. Utilize behavioral rehearsal and role play of peer group interaction to teach the client social skills and reduce social anxiety.

12. Encourage the client to invite a friend for an overnight visit and/or set up an overnight visit at a friend's home; process any fears that arise and reinforce independence.

13. Assign the client a task (e.g., a special chore at home, writing a school paper on a topic of interest) that facilitates autonomy and reinforces confidence and a sense of empowerment.

14. Require the client to perform a ritual at night (e.g., reassuringly put a stuffed animal or doll to bed, read a story with a parent, place a bad-dream catcher in the room) to manage fears and facilitate autonomy.

15. Refocus the client's discussion from physical complaints to emotional conflicts and the expression of feelings.

16. Assist the client and his/her parents in developing insight into the secondary

18. Identify and express feelings connected with a past separation, loss, or trauma. (28, 30, 31, 33, 34)

19. Increase the frequency of positive self-descriptive statements. (6, 13, 27)

20. Increase assertive behaviors to deal more effectively and directly with stress, conflict, or responsibilities. (11, 13, 25)

21. Increase communication and intimacy between the parents. (17, 23, 25, 35)

22. Take prescribed medication as directed by the physician. (36, 37, 38)

—. _____
   _____

—. _____
   _____

—. _____
   _____

gain received from physical illnesses, complaints, and the like.

17. Conduct family therapy sessions to assess the dynamics contributing to the emergence of the client's separation anxiety and fears.

18. Utilize a family-sculpting technique, in which the client defines the role and behavior of each family member in a scene of his/her choosing to assess family dynamics.

19. Identify how the enmeshed or overly protective parent(s) reinforce the client's dependency and irrational fears.

20. Encourage the parents to reinforce the client's autonomous behaviors (e.g., independent play, socializing with friends) and set limits on overly dependent behaviors (e.g., insisting that the parent be in the same room, going into the parents' room at night).

21. Counsel the parents about setting firm, consistent limits on the client's temper tantrums and excessive clinging or whining.

22. Give a directive to the disengaged or distant parent to spend more time or perform a specific task with the client (e.g., work on a project around the home, assist the client with homework, go on an outing together).

23. Assess the marital dyad for possible conflict and triangulation of the client into discord.

24. Use a paradoxical intervention (e.g., instruct the client and his/her parent to tie a six-foot string to each other every day so they can never be separated) to work around the family's resistance and disengage the client from overly protective parent(s).

25. Counsel family members about the need for appropriate boundaries, space, and privacy.

26. Assess whether the client's anxiety and fears are associated with a separation, loss, trauma, or realistic danger.

27. Actively build the level of trust with the client in individual sessions through consistent eye contact, active listening, unconditional positive regard, and warm acceptance to help him/her increase the ability to identify and express feelings.

28. Explore, encourage, and support the client in verbally expressing and clarifying the feelings associated with the separation, loss, trauma, or realistic danger.

29. Identify and implement the steps necessary to protect the client from ongoing danger or trauma.

30. Assign the client to write a letter to express his/her feelings about a past separation, loss, trauma, or danger; process the letter with the therapist.

31. Request that the client perform a letting-go exercise in which a symbol of a past separation, loss, or trauma is destroyed; process this with the therapist.

32. Assist the client in differentiating between realistic and unrealistic fears.

33. Utilize individual play therapy sessions to provide the client with the opportunity to express and work through his/her feelings and fears.

34. Interpret the feelings and fears expressed in play therapy and relate them to the client's present life situation.

35. Teach effective communication skills to the client and his/her parent(s).

36. Arrange for psychotropic medication for the client, if necessary.

37. Monitor the client for compliance, side effects, and overall effectiveness of the medication.

38. Refer the client for a medical examination to rule out genuine health problems.

—. _____
   _____

—. _____
   _____

—. _____
   _____

DIAGNOSTIC SUGGESTIONS

Axis I: 309.21   Separation Anxiety
               300.02   Generalized Anxiety Disorder
               300.23   Social Phobia
               296.xx   Major Depressive Disorder
               300.82   Somatization Disorder
               301.47   Nightmare Disorder
               307.46   Sleep Terror Disorder
               309.81   Posttraumatic Stress Disorder

               _____   _____
               _____   _____

Axis II: 799.9   Diagnosis Deferred
               V71.09   No Diagnosis

               _____   _____
               _____   _____

SEXUAL ABUSE PERPETRATOR

BEHAVIORAL DEFINITIONS

1. Arrest and conviction for a sexually related crime such as exhibitionism, exposure, voyeurism, fondling, statutory rape, or criminal sexual misconduct (first, second, third degree).
2. Client's language has an easily noted sexual content.
3. Evident sexualization to most, if not all, relationships.
4. Focus on and preoccupation with anything of a sexual nature.
5. Positive familial history for incest.

—. _____
   _____
—. _____
   _____
—. _____
   _____

LONG-TERM GOALS

1. Eliminate all inappropriate sexual behaviors.
2. Establish and honor boundaries that reflect a sense of mutual respect in all interpersonal relationships.
3. Become capable of forming nonsexual relationships.
4. Reach the point of genuine self-forgiveness and ask for forgiveness from the violated individual(s) along with making an offer of restitution.
5. Acknowledge and take responsibility for all inappropriate sexual behavior.
6. Resolve issues of his/her own sexual abuse.

—. _____
   _____
   _____
—. _____
   _____
   _____
—. _____
   _____

SHORT-TERM OBJECTIVES

1. Develop a working relationship with the therapist in which the client shares his/her thoughts and feelings openly. (1, 2, 3)

2. Verbally agree to and sign a no-sexual-contact agreement. (1, 4, 5, 6)

3. Increase the verbal acknowledgment of the abuse and responsibility for his/her actions regarding it. (1, 3, 7, 8)

4. Recognize and honor the personal boundaries of others as shown by the termination of inappropriate sexual contact. (8, 9, 10, 11)

5. Decrease the frequency of sexual references in daily speech and sexual actions in daily behavior. (1, 8, 12, 13)

6. Provide a complete sexual history. (1, 14)

THERAPEUTIC INTERVENTIONS

1. Actively build the level of trust with the client in individual sessions through consistent eye contact, active listening, unconditional positive regard, and warm acceptance to help increase his/her ability to identify and express feelings.

2. Use a celebrity interview format in which the client is asked nonthreatening questions such as his/her likes and dislikes, best times, favorite holidays, and so on, to initiate self-disclosure.

3. Use a therapeutic game (Talking, Feeling, Doing* or The Ungame†) to start the client talking about him/herself and to expand the client's self-awareness.

4. Work with the client and his/her family to develop

---

* Creative Therapeutics, Cresskill, New Jersey, 1973.
† The Ungame Co., Anaheim, California, 1984.

7. Verbally acknowledge any incidence of sexual abuse. (1, 3, 15, 16)

8. Tell the story of the abuse with appropriate affect. (1, 17, 18, 19, 20)

9. Increase the ability to identify and express feelings. (3, 20, 21, 22)

10. Identify irrational thoughts, feelings, and beliefs that give justification for sexual abuse. (8, 19, 23)

11. Increase the formation of positive peer relationships. (22, 24, 25, 27)

12. Practice the SAFE method (avoiding a relationship if there is anything Secret about it, if it is Abusive to oneself or others, if it is used to avoid Feelings, or if it is Empty of caring and commitment) when relating with others. (3, 22, 29)

13. Make an apology to the survivor and the family, which includes an offer of restitution. (22, 30, 31)

14. Increase the family's awareness of the patterns, beliefs, and behaviors that support the client's sexual behavior. (19, 32, 33, 34)

15. The parents identify key changes the family will need to make to assist in the client's recovery and begin to implement these changes. (32, 33, 34, 25)

and implement a behaviorally specific no-sexual-contact agreement.

5. Monitor, along with the parents, the client's no-sexual-contact agreement, making adjustments as necessary and giving both positive and negative feedback as warranted.

6. Refer the client to a more appropriate restrictive setting if the no-sexual-contact agreement is violated.

7. Process the behavior and incidents of sexual misconduct and/or abuse, focusing on getting the whole story out and having the client accept responsibility for his/her behavior.

8. Refer the client to a group for sexual perpetrators.

9. Educate the client about appropriate and inappropriate sexual behavior.

10. Assist the client in becoming aware of personal sexual boundaries and how to respect and honor them.

11. Role-play social situations in which sexual boundaries are involved. Give the client feedback on his/her actions and model appropriate behavior.

12. Point out to the client sexual references and content in his/her speech and behavior. Process the feelings and thoughts that underlie the references.

16. Develop and implement an aftercare plan for the client that includes the support of the family. (35, 36, 37, 38)

17. Complete psychological testing and receive the results. (1, 39, 40)

18. Comply with any investigations by child protective services or criminal justice officials. (1, 41, 42)

__. _____
_____

__. _____
_____

__. _____
_____

13. Ask the client to gather feedback from teachers, parents, and so on, regarding sexual references in his/her speech and behavior. Process the feedback with the client and look at alternatives.

14. Gather a thorough sexual history of the client from both the client and his/her parents.

15. Gently probe whether the client was sexually abused by asking specific questions regarding others' respect for the client's physical boundaries when he/she was a child.

16. Assist the client in identifying the consequences of his/her sexual abuse in the development of his/her own attitudes and patterns of behavior.

17. Encourage and support the client in telling the story of his/her abuse.

18. Prepare, assist, and support the client in telling his/her parents of the abuse.

19. Conduct a family session in which a genogram is developed that depicts patterns of interaction and identifies family members who are sexual abuse survivors or perpetrators, or have been involved in other sexual deviancy.

20. Refer the client to a group for survivors of sexual abuse.

21. Assist the client in becoming capable of identifying and expressing his/her feelings.

22. Give feedback to the client when he/she does not show awareness of the feelings of him/herself or others and positive verbal reinforcement when he/she does so without direction.

23. Assist the client in identifying thoughts and beliefs that gave justification for the abuse. Then work to replace them with socially acceptable ones that are respectful and not exploitive of others.

24. Help the client identify specific ways he/she can become more involved with peers.

25. Role-play various peer social situations to help the client become more comfortable and confident in interactions.

26. Ask the client to attempt one new social or recreational activity each week. Process the experience.

27. Assign the client to engage a peer in conversation and/or an appropriate play activity once daily. Process the results with the therapist in the weekly session.

28. Refer the client to an experiential camp that focuses on increasing interpersonal skills with peers and individual self-confidence.

29. Teach the client the SAFE
     formula (see Objective #12)
     for relationships. Monitor
     his/her use and give feed-
     back and redirection as
     required.

30. Assist the client in reaching
     the point where he/she is
     ready to make a genuine
     apology for the behavior.
     Then prepare the client to
     do so face to face with the
     survivor.

31. Conduct a family session
     with both the perpetrator's
     and the survivor's families
     in which the perpetrator
     apologizes to the survivor
     and his/her family and
     some form of restitution is
     worked out.

32. Hold family sessions that
     explore sexual patterns,
     beliefs, and behaviors. Then
     assist the family members
     in identifying what sexual
     patterns, beliefs, or behav-
     iors need to be changed and
     how they can begin to
     change them.

33. Conduct family sessions in
     which structural interven-
     tions are developed and
     implemented by the family
     (e.g., family members begin
     closing doors within their
     home or remove children
     from roles as supervisors of
     other siblings).

34. Where there is a noncusto-
     dial or distant parent of the
     same sex, hold family ses-

sions in which the strategic intervention is implemented of placing this parent in charge of the client's sexual education and monitoring his/her sexual behavior.

35. Refer the client's parents to a support group for parents of perpetrators or to parenting classes.

36. Ask the client and his/her family to develop a written aftercare plan. Process the plan in a family session and make adjustments as necessary.

37. Request that the client and his/her family commit to periodic checkups with the therapist as part of an aftercare plan.

38. Hold checkup sessions in which the aftercare plan is reviewed for effectiveness and follow-through. Give feedback and make adjustments as necessary.

39. Arrange for psychological testing to rule out severe emotional issues or psychopathology.

40. Present and interpret the results of psychological testing. Emphasize the recommendations as they apply to ongoing treatment and answer any questions the client has.

41. Report any sexual abuse that is revealed by the client to child protective services or appropriate criminal justice officials.

42. Ask the client to tell the therapist the outcome of the investigation and then process the results in a session focusing on the issues of taking responsibility for his/her behavior and respecting the personal boundaries of others.

___. _____
_____

___. _____
_____

___. _____
_____

DIAGNOSTIC SUGGESTIONS

Axis I:	312.81	Conduct Disorder/Childhood-Onset Type
	312.82	Conduct Disorder/Adolescent-Onset Type
	302.2	Pedophilia
	302.4	Exhibitionism
	302.82	Voyeurism
	V61.8	Sibling Relational Problem
	V61.21	Sexual Abuse of Child
	V71.02	Child or Adolescent Antisocial Behavior
	_____	_____
	_____	_____
Axis II:	799.9	Diagnosis Deferred
	V71.09	No Diagnosis
	_____	_____
	_____	_____

SEXUAL ABUSE VICTIM

BEHAVIORAL DEFINITIONS

1. Self-report of being sexually abused.
2. Physical signs of sexual abuse (e.g., red or swollen genitalia, blood in the underwear, constant rashes, a tear in the vagina or rectum, venereal disease, hickeys on the body).
3. Strong interest in or curiosity about advanced knowledge of sexuality.
4. Sexual themes or sexualized behaviors emerge in play or art work.
5. Sexualized or seductive behavior with younger children, peers, or adults (e.g., provocative exhibition of genitalia, fondling, mutual masturbation, anal or vaginal penetration).
6. Recurrent and intrusive distressing recollections or nightmares of the abuse.
7. Acting or feeling as if the sexual abuse were recurring (including delusions, hallucinations, dissociative flashback experiences).
8. Unexplainable feelings of anger, rage, or fear when coming into contact with the perpetrator or after exposure to sexual topics.
9. Pronounced disturbance of mood and affect (i.e., frequent and prolonged periods of depression, irritability, anxiety, and fearfulness).
10. Appearance of regressive behaviors (e.g., thumb sucking, baby talk, bed-wetting).
11. Marked distrust in others as manifested by social withdrawal and difficulty in maintaining close relationships.

—. _____

_____

—. _____

_____

—. _____

_____

LONG-TERM GOALS

1. Cease all further sexual victimization of the client.
2. Work successfully through the issue of sexual abuse with consequent understanding and control of feelings and behavior.
3. Resolve the issues surrounding the sexual abuse, resulting in an ability to establish and maintain close interpersonal relationships.
4. Establish appropriate boundaries and generational lines in the family to greatly minimize the risk of sexual abuse ever occurring in the future.
5. Achieve healing within the family system as evidenced by the verbal expression of forgiveness and a willingness to let go and move on.
6. Eliminate denial in the client and the family, placing responsibility for the abuse on the perpetrator and allowing the survivor to feel supported.
7. Eliminate all inappropriate sexual behaviors.
8. Build self-esteem and a sense of empowerment in the client as manifested by an increased number of positive self-descriptive statements and greater participation in extracurricular activities.

—. _____
_____
_____

—. _____
_____
_____

—. _____
_____

SHORT-TERM OBJECTIVES	THERAPEUTIC INTERVENTIONS
1. Tell the entire story of the abuse. (1, 2, 3, 6, 18, 31)	1. Actively build the level of trust with the client in individual sessions through consistent eye contact, active listening, unconditional positive regard, and warm acceptance to help increase his/her ability to identify and express feelings.
2. Identify the nature, frequency, and duration of the abuse. (1, 2, 3, 4, 6)	
3. Identify and express feelings connected to the abuse. (1, 2, 17, 25, 27)	
4. Decrease secrecy in the family by informing key members about the abuse. (6, 10, 16, 21)	2. Explore, encourage, and support the client in ver-

5. Verbally demonstrate a knowledge of sexual abuse and its effects. (12, 14, 17, 24)

6. Verbalize the way sexual abuse has impacted his/her life. (2, 24, 25)

7. Verbally identify the perpetrator as being responsible for the sexual abuse. (10, 17, 20, 21, 26)

8. Decrease expressed feelings of shame and guilt and affirm him/herself as not being responsible for the abuse. (2, 17, 20, 25, 30)

9. Increase the openness to talk about sexual abuse in the family. (6, 10, 14, 16, 34)

10. Stabilize the mood and decrease the emotional intensity connected to the abuse. (2, 8, 11, 12, 16)

11. Increase support and acceptance from the nonabusive parent and other key family members. (10, 13, 14, 16, 32)

12. Establish appropriate boundaries between the client and his/her parent(s) to ensure protection. (7, 8, 9, 13, 14)

13. Establish and adhere to appropriate intimacy boundaries within the family. (8, 13, 14, 15, 33)

14. Decrease the statements of being a victim while increasing statements that reflect personal empowerment. (12, 19, 23, 24)

bally expressing and clarifying his/her feelings associated with the abuse.

3. Report sexual abuse to the appropriate child protection agency, criminal justice officials, or medical professionals.

4. Consult with a physician, criminal justice officials, or child protection case managers to assess the veracity of the sexual abuse charges.

5. Consult with a physician, criminal justice officials, and child protection case managers to develop appropriate treatment interventions.

6. Facilitate conjoint sessions to reveal the sexual abuse to key family member(s) or caregiver(s).

7. Assess whether the perpetrator should be removed from the home.

8. Implement the necessary steps to protect the client and other children in the home from future sexual abuse.

9. Assess whether the client is safe to remain in the home or should be removed.

10. Actively confront and challenge denial within the family system.

11. Arrange for a medication evaluation.

12. Empower the client by reinforcing the steps necessary to protect him/herself.

15. Terminate the client's verbalizations of excuses for the perpetrator. (10, 17, 25)

16. Increase the client's level of forgiveness of the perpetrator and others connected with the abuse. (17, 19, 20, 23)

17. Verbally self-identify as a survivor of sexual abuse. (23, 24, 25)

18. Increase the level of trust of others as shown by increased socialization and a greater number of friendships. (22, 25, 29)

19. Increase outside family contacts and social networks. (22, 25, 26, 29)

20. Have the perpetrator take responsibility for the abuse. (7, 20, 21, 26)

21. Have the perpetrator ask for the client's forgiveness and pledge respect for boundaries. (19, 20)

22. Have the perpetrator agree to seek treatment. (3, 5, 21, 26, 33)

—. _____
_____

—. _____
_____

—. _____
_____

13. Counsel the client's family member(s) about appropriate boundaries.

14. Assess the family dynamics and identify the stress factors or precipitating events that contributed to the emergence of the abuse.

15. Evaluate the possibility of substance abuse problems within the client's family.

16. Elicit and reinforce support and nurturance for the client from other key family member(s).

17. Assign the client to write a letter to the perpetrator and process it with the therapist.

18. Assign the client to draw a diagram of the house where the abuse occurred, indicating where everyone slept, and share the diagram with the therapist.

19. Assign the client to write a forgiveness letter and/or complete a forgiveness exercise in which he/she verbalizes forgiveness to the perpetrator and/or significant family member(s). Process this with the therapist.

20. Hold a session where the perpetrator apologizes to the client and/or other family member(s).

21. Hold a therapy session where the client and/or the therapist confront the perpetrator with the abuse.

22. Teach the client the share-check method of building trust, in which the degree of shared information is related to a proven level of trustworthiness.

23. Assign the client a letting-go exercise in which a symbol of the abuse is disposed of or destroyed. Process this with the therapist.

24. Ask the client to identify the positive and negative consequences of being a victim versus being a survivor. Compare and process the lists with the therapist.

25. Refer the client to a survivor support group with other children to assist them in realizing that they are not alone in having experienced sexual abuse.

26. Require the perpetrator to participate in a sexual offenders group.

27. Utilize individual play therapy sessions to provide the client with the opportunity to express and work through feelings.

28. Arrange for psychological testing with the client and/or family member(s) to rule out the presence of severe psychological disorders.

29. Encourage the client to participate in positive peer groups or extracurricular activities.

30. Assign the client to read *A Very Touching Book* (Hindman), *I Can't Talk About It* (Sanford), or *It's Not Your Fault* (Jance); process the concepts with the therapist.

31. Use anatomically detailed dolls to have the client tell and show how he/she was abused. Take great caution not to lead the client.

32. Assign the client's parents and significant others to read *Allies in Healing* (Davis) to assist them in understanding how they can help.

33. Assign the client's family to read *Out of the Shadows* (Carnes) to expand their knowledge of sexually addictive behaviors.

34. Construct a multigenerational family genogram that identifies sexual abuse within the extended family to help the client realize that he/she is not the only one abused and to help the perpetrator recognize the cycle of boundary violation.

___. _____

_____

___. _____

_____

___. _____

_____

DIAGNOSTIC SUGGESTIONS

Axis I:	309.81	Posttraumatic Stress Disorder
	308.3	Acute Stress Disorder
	296.xx	Major Depressive Disorder
	309.21	Separation Anxiety Disorder
	V61.21	Sexual Abuse of Child, 995.53 Victim
	307.47	Nightmare Disorder
	300.6	Depersonalization Disorder
	300.15	Dissociative Disorder NOS
	_____	_____
	_____	_____
Axis II:	799.9	Diagnosis Deferred
	V71.09	No Diagnosis
	_____	_____
	_____	_____

SLEEP DISTURBANCE

BEHAVIORAL DEFINITIONS

1. Emotional distress (e.g., crying, leaving bed to awaken the parents, demanding to sleep with the parents) that accompanies difficulty falling asleep or maintaining sleep.
2. Difficulty getting to or maintaining sleep without significant demands made on the parents.
3. Distress (e.g., crying, calling for the parents, the heart racing, or fear of returning to sleep) resulting from repeated awakening with detailed recall of extremely frightening dreams involving threats to him/herself or significant others.
4. Repeated incidents of leaving bed and walking about in an apparent sleep state but the eyes are open, the face is blank, there is no response to communication efforts, and amnesia for the incident upon awakening.
5. Abrupt awakening with a panicky scream followed by intense anxiety and autonomic arousal, no detailed dream recall, and unresponsiveness to the efforts of others to give comfort during the episode.
6. Irresistible, involuntary attacks of sleep that occur daily during times of normal wakefulness, accompanied by a bilateral loss of muscle tone and/or REM sleep dreams or paralysis at the beginning or end of the sleep episodes.
7. Insomnia or hypersomnia complaints due to a reversal of the sleep-wake schedule normal for the client's environment.
8. Prolonged sleep and/or excessive daytime napping that does not result in feeling adequately rested or refreshed but continually tired.

__. _____

_____

__. _____
    _____
__. _____
    _____

LONG-TERM GOALS

1. Fall asleep calmly and stays asleep without an undue, reassuring parental presence required.
2. Feel refreshed and energetic during wakeful hours.
3. Cease anxiety-producing dreams that cause awakening.
4. End abrupt awakening in terror and return to a peaceful, restful sleep pattern.
5. Restore restful sleep with a reduction of sleepwalking incidents.

__. _____
    _____
__. _____
    _____
__. _____
    _____

SHORT-TERM OBJECTIVES

1. Identify daily stressors and the associated sleep patterns. (1, 6, 11)

2. Verbalize depressive feelings and share the possible causes. (2, 5, 6, 15, 16)

3. Describe experiences of emotional trauma that continue to disturb sleep. (3, 5, 6, 7, 8)

4. Describe disturbing dreams. (1, 3, 4)

THERAPEUTIC INTERVENTIONS

1. Assess the role of daily stressors in the interruption of the client's sleep.

2. Assess the role of depression as a cause of the client's sleep disturbances.

3. Explore recent traumatic events that interfere with the client's sleep.

4. Probe the nature of the client's disturbing dreams and their relationship to life stress.

5. Reveal sexual abuse incidents that continue to be disturbing.

6. Remain alone in the bedroom without expressions of fear. (5, 6, 7, 8, 9)

7. Follow a sleep-induction schedule of events. (9, 10, 13)

8. The parents develop a practice of setting firm limits on the client's manipulatory behavior. (9, 10, 13)

9. The parents identify sources of conflict or stress within the marriage and family. (11, 12)

10. The parents verbalize the resolution of conflict within the family. (11, 12)

11. The parents consistently adhere to a bedtime routine as developed in a family therapy session. (13)

12. The client and his/her parents cooperate with obtaining a physical exam for the client. (14)

13. Take psychotropic medication as prescribed to assess its effect on sleep. (2, 3, 15, 16)

14. Practice deep-muscle relaxation exercises. (17, 18)

15. Utilize biofeedback training to deepen relaxation skills. (17, 18)

5. Explore the possibility of sexual abuse to the client that has not been revealed.

6. Utilize play therapy techniques to assess and resolve emotional conflicts.

7. Interpret the client's play behavior as reflective of his/her feelings toward family members.

8. Assess the client's fears associated with being alone in the bedroom in terms of their nature, severity, and origin.

9. Confront the client's irrational fears and teach cognitive strategies (e.g., positive, realistic self-talk) to reduce them.

10. Meet with the parents to help them set firm limits on the client's manipulative bedtime behavior.

11. Meet with the family to assess the level of tension and conflict and its effect on the client's sleep.

12. Hold family therapy sessions to resolve conflicts and reduce the tension level in the home.

13. Meet with the client and his/her parents to establish a bedtime routine that is calming and attentive but consistent and firm. Involve the client in the development process.

16. Share a history of substance abuse or medication use and, if necessary, assume responsibility for the chemical dependence problem. (19)

__. _____

_____

__. _____

_____

__. _____

_____

14. Refer the client to a physician to rule out any physical and pharmacological causes for the sleep disturbance.

15. Arrange for antidepressant medication for the client to enhance restful sleep.

16. Monitor the client for medication compliance and effectiveness.

17. Train the client in deep-muscle relaxation exercises with and without audiotape instruction.

18. Administer electromyographic (EMG) biofeedback to reinforce the successful relaxation response.

19. Assess the contribution of medication or substance abuse to the client's sleep disorder and, if necessary, treat the chemical dependence problem.

__. _____

_____

__. _____

_____

__. _____

_____

DIAGNOSTIC SUGGESTIONS

Axis I:	309.21	Separation Anxiety Disorder, Early Onset
	312.9	Disruptive Behavior Disorder NOS
	307.42	Primary Insomnia
	307.44	Primary Hypersomnia
	307.45	Circadian Rhythm Sleep Disorder
	307.47	Nightmare Disorder
	307.46	Sleep Terror Disorder
	307.46	Sleepwalking Disorder
	309.81	Posttraumatic Stress Disorder
	296.xx	Major Depressive Disorder
	300.4	Dysthymic Disorder
	296.xx	Bipolar I Disorder
	296.89	Bipolar II Disorder
	296.80	Bipolar Disorder NOS
	301.13	Cyclothymic Disorder
	_____	_____
	_____	_____
Axis II:	799.9	Diagnosis Deferred
	V71.09	No Diagnosis
	_____	_____
	_____	_____

SOCIAL PHOBIA/SHYNESS

BEHAVIORAL DEFINITIONS

1. Hiding, limited or no eye contact, a refusal or reticence to respond verbally to overtures from others, and isolation in most social situations.
2. Excessive shrinking or avoidance of contact with unfamiliar people for an extended period of time (i.e., six months or longer).
3. Social isolation and/or excessive involvement in isolated activities (e.g., reading, listening to music in his/her room, playing video games).
4. Extremely limited or no close friendships outside the immediate family members.
5. Hypersensitivity to criticism or disapproval by others.
6. Excessive need for reassurance that he/she is liked by others before demonstrating a willingness to get involved with other people.
7. Marked reluctance to engage in new activities or take personal risks because of the potential for embarrassment or humiliation.
8. Negative self-image as evidenced by frequent self-disparaging remarks, unfavorable comparisons to others, and a perception of him/herself as being socially unattractive.
9. Lack of assertiveness because of a fear of being met with criticism, disapproval, or rejection.
10. Heightened physiological distress in social settings as manifested by increased heart rate, profuse sweating, dry mouth, muscular tension, and trembling.

__. _____

_____

__. _____

_____

—. _____

_____

LONG-TERM GOALS

1. Eliminate anxiety, shyness, and timidity in most social settings.
2. Establish and maintain long-term (i.e., six months) interpersonal relationships or peer friendships outside of the immediate family.
3. Interact socially with peers or friends on a regular, consistent basis without excessive fear or anxiety.
4. Achieve a healthy balance between time spent in solitary activity and social interaction with others.
5. Develop the essential social skills that will enhance the quality of interpersonal relationships.
6. Resolve the core conflicts contributing to the emergence of social anxiety and shyness.
7. Elevate the self-esteem and feelings of security in interpersonal relationships as evidenced by a willingness to participate in peer group activities and express thoughts, feelings, and needs on a regular basis.

—. _____

_____

—. _____

_____

—. _____

_____

SHORT-TERM OBJECTIVES

1. Complete psychological testing. (1, 4)
2. Complete psychoeducational testing. (2, 4)
3. Complete a speech/language evaluation. (3, 4)
4. Comply with the behavioral and cognitive strategies and

THERAPEUTIC INTERVENTIONS

1. Arrange for psychological testing to assess the severity of the client's anxiety and gain greater insight into the dynamics contributing to the symptoms.
2. Arrange for psychoeducational testing of the client to

gradually increase the frequency and duration of social contacts. (5, 6, 7, 8, 9)

5. Agree to initiate one social contact per day. (6, 8, 12, 14, 15)

6. Increase participation in interpersonal or peer group activities. (11, 12, 13, 14, 15)

7. Increase the verbalizations of positive statements about him/herself, peer interactions, and social experiences. (11, 12, 13, 14, 16)

8. Verbally acknowledge compliments without excessive timidity or withdrawal. (9, 10, 16, 17)

9. Increase positive self-statements in social interactions. (9, 10, 17)

10. Decrease the frequency of self-disparaging remarks in the presence of peers. (8, 9, 16, 17, 18)

11. Increase assertive behaviors to deal more effectively and directly with stress, conflict, and responsibilities. (17, 18, 28, 29)

12. The enmeshed or overly protective parent(s) identify how they reinforce social anxiety and overly dependent behaviors. (22, 24, 25, 27)

13. Verbally recognize the secondary gain that results from social anxiety, self-disparaging remarks, and overdependence on the parents. (22, 25, 27)

rule out the presence of a learning disability.

3. Refer the client for a comprehensive, speech/language evaluation to rule out possible impairment that may contribute to social withdrawal.

4. Give feedback to the client and his/her family regarding psychological and psychoeducational testing.

5. Design and implement a systematic desensitization program in which the client gradually increases the frequency and duration of social contacts to help decrease his/her social anxiety.

6. Assign the task of initiating one social contact per day.

7. Train the client to reduce anxiety utilizing guided imagery in a relaxed state with the client visualizing him/herself dealing with various social situations in a confident manner.

8. Assist the client in developing positive self-talk as a means of managing his/her social anxiety or fears.

9. Utilize behavioral rehearsal, modeling, and role play in individual sessions to reduce anxiety, develop social skills, and learn to initiate conversation.

10. Praise and reinforce any emerging positive social behaviors.

14. The parents reinforce the client's positive social behaviors and set limits on overly dependent behaviors. (14, 24, 25, 26)

15. The overly critical parent(s) verbally recognize how their negative remarks contribute to the client's social anxiety, timidity, and low self-esteem. (22, 23, 26)

16. The parents set realistic and age-appropriate goals for the client. (22, 23, 26)

17. Verbalize how current social anxiety and insecurities are associated with past rejection experiences and criticism from significant others. (19, 20, 21)

18. Take medication as directed by the prescribing physician. (30, 31)

__. _____
   _____
__. _____
   _____
__. _____
   _____

11. Ask the client to list how he/she is like his/her peers.

12. Encourage participation in extracurricular or positive peer group activities.

13. Ask the client to list or keep a journal of both positive and negative social experiences; process this with the therapist.

14. Give the client a directive to invite a friend for an overnight visit and/or set up an overnight visit at a friend's home; process any fears and anxiety that arise.

15. Consult with school officials about ways to increase the client's socialization (e.g., give a presentation to the class in an area of interest or expertise, tutor a more popular peer, pair the client with another popular peer on classroom assignments).

16. Provide feedback on any negative social behaviors that interfere with the client's ability to establish and maintain friendships.

17. Teach assertiveness skills to help the client communicate thoughts, feelings, and needs more openly and directly.

18. Explore for a history of rejection experiences, harsh criticism, abandonment, or trauma that fostered the client's low self-esteem and social anxiety.

19. Encourage and support the client in verbally expressing and clarifying his/her feelings associated with past rejection experiences, harsh criticism, abandonment, or trauma.

20. Utilize individual play therapy sessions to provide the client with the opportunity to express and work through his/her anxiety and feelings of insecurity surrounding social relationships.

21. Interpret the anxiety and insecurity expressed in play therapy and relate them to the client's present life situations.

22. Conduct a family therapy session to assess the dynamics contributing to the client's social anxiety and withdrawal.

23. Assess the parent-child dyad to determine whether the parent(s) place unrealistically high standards on the client that contribute to the anxiety and feelings of insecurity.

24. Identify how the overly protective parent(s) reinforce the client's dependency and social anxiety.

25. Encourage the parents to reinforce or reward the client's positive social behaviors (e.g., calling a friend, playing with peers outside the home) and set

limits on overly dependent behaviors (e.g., pleading, clinging to the parents in social settings).

26. Instruct the parents to ignore occasional and mild antisocial or aggressive behaviors by the client (unless they become too intense or frequent) during the initial stages of treatment so as not to extinguish emerging assertive behaviors.

27. Assist the client and his/her parent(s) in developing insight into the secondary gain received from social anxiety and withdrawal.

28. Arrange for the client to attend group therapy to improve his/her social skills.

29. Give the client a directive to self-disclose two times in each group therapy session.

30. Arrange for a medication evaluation of the client.

31. Monitor the client for compliance, side effects, and overall effectiveness of the medication. Consult with the prescribing physician at regular intervals.

__. _____
    _____

__. _____
    _____

__. _____
    _____

DIAGNOSTIC SUGGESTIONS

Axis I: 300.23   Social Phobia
                300.02   Generalized Anxiety Disorder
                300.00   Anxiety Disorder NOS
                309.21   Separation Anxiety
                300.4   Dysthymic Disorder
                296.xx   Major Depressive Disorder
                311   Depressive Disorder NOS
                309.81   Posttraumatic Stress Disorder

                _____   _____

                _____   _____

Axis II: 799.9   Diagnosis Deferred
                V71.09   No Diagnosis

                _____   _____

                _____   _____

SPEECH/LANGUAGE DISORDERS

BEHAVIORAL DEFINITIONS

1. Expressive language abilities, as measured by standardized tests, substantially below the expected level.
2. Expressive language deficits, as demonstrated by markedly limited vocabulary, frequent errors in tense, and difficulty recalling words or producing sentences of developmentally appropriate length or complexity.
3. Receptive and expressive language abilities, as measured by standardized tests, significantly below the expected level.
4. Receptive language deficits, as manifested by difficulty understanding simple words or sentences, certain types of words such as spatial terms, or longer, complex statements.
5. Deficits in expressive and/or receptive language development that significantly interfere with academic or occupational achievement or with social communication.
6. Consistent failure to use or produce developmentally expected speech sounds.
7. Repeated stuttering as demonstrated by impairment in the normal fluency and time patterning of speech.
8. Deficits in speech sound production or fluency that significantly interfere with academic or occupational achievement or with social communication.
9. Selective mutism as characterized by a consistent failure to speak in specific social situations (e.g., school) despite speaking in other situations.
10. Social withdrawal and isolation in the peer group, school, or social settings where the individual may be required to speak.
11. Recurrent pattern of engaging in acting-out, aggressive, or negative attention-seeking behaviors when encountering frustration with speech or language problems.

—. _____
   _____
   _____
—. _____
   _____
   _____
—. _____
   _____

LONG-TERM GOALS

1. Achieve the speech and language goals identified in the Individualized Educational Plan (IEP).
2. Improve the expressive and receptive language abilities to the level of capability.
3. Achieve mastery of the expected speech sounds that are appropriate for the age and dialect.
4. Eliminate stuttering; speak fluently and at a normal rate on a regular, consistent basis.
5. Develop an awareness and acceptance of speech/language problems so that there is consistent participation in discussions in the peer group, school, or social settings.
6. The parents establish realistic expectations of their child's speech/language abilities.
7. Resolve the core conflict that contributes to the emergence of selective mutism so that the client speaks consistently in all social situations.
8. Eliminate the pattern of engaging in acting-out, aggressive, or negative attention-seeking behaviors when experiencing the frustration associated with speech/language problems.

—. _____
   _____
—. _____
   _____
—. _____
   _____

SHORT-TERM OBJECTIVES

1. Complete a speech/language evaluation to determine eligibility for special education services. (1, 6)

2. Complete a psychoeducational evaluation. (2, 6)

3. Complete psychological testing. (3, 6)

4. Complete neuropsychological testing. (4, 6)

5. Cooperate with a hearing or medical examination. (1, 5, 6)

6. Cease verbalizations of denial in the family system about the client's speech/language problem. (6, 7, 11, 12)

7. Comply with the recommendations made by a multidisciplinary evaluation team at school regarding speech/language or educational interventions. (6, 7, 8)

8. Verbalize an acceptance of appropriate special education services to address the speech/language deficits. (6, 7, 8, 12)

9. Comply with speech therapy and cooperate with the recommendations or interventions offered by the speech/language pathologist. (6, 7, 8, 9, 12)

10. The parents, teachers, and speech/language pathologist implement interventions that maximize the client's

THERAPEUTIC INTERVENTIONS

1. Refer the client for a speech/language evaluation to assess the presence of a disorder and determine his/her eligibility for special education services.

2. Arrange for a psychoeducational evaluation to assess the client's intellectual abilities and rule out the presence of other possible learning disabilities.

3. Arrange for psychological testing to determine whether emotional factors or ADHD are interfering with the client's speech/language development.

4. Arrange for a neurological examination or neuropsychological evaluation to rule out the presence of organic factors that may contribute to the client's speech/language problem.

5. Refer the client for a hearing or medical examination to rule out problems that may be interfering with his/her speech/language development.

6. Attend an IEP committee meeting with the client's parents, teachers, and the speech/language pathologist to determine his/her eligibility for special education services, design educational interventions, establish speech/language goals, and

strengths and compensate for impairments. (6, 7, 9, 11, 12)

11. The parents maintain regular communication with teachers and the speech/language pathologist. (7, 8, 9, 11)

12. Increase praise and positive reinforcement by the parents toward the client in regard to speech/language development. (7, 10, 13, 14, 22)

13. Increase the time spent between the client and his/her parents in activities that build and facilitate speech/language development. (13, 14)

14. The parents recognize and verbally acknowledge their unrealistic expectations for or excessive pressure on the client to develop speech/language abilities. (15, 16, 17)

15. The parents recognize and verbally acknowledge their tendency to speak for the client in social settings. (7, 18, 19, 20)

16. The parents cease their pattern of speaking for the client in social settings where it is not appropriate. (17, 18, 19, 20)

17. Improve the lines of communication in the family system. (17, 19, 20)

18. Increase the frequency of social interactions in which the client takes the lead in

outline emotional issues to deal with in counseling.

7. Consult with the client, his/her parents, teachers, and the speech/language pathologist about designing effective intervention strategies that build on the client's strengths and compensate for weaknesses.

8. Refer the client to a private speech/language pathologist for extra assistance in improving speech/language abilities.

9. Encourage the parents to maintain regular communication with his/her teachers and the speech/language pathologist to help facilitate the client's speech/language development.

10. Encourage the parents to give frequent praise and positive reinforcement regarding the client's speech/language development.

11. Educate the parents about the signs and symptoms of the client's speech/language disorder.

12. Challenge the parents' denial surrounding the client's speech/language problem so that the parents cooperate with the recommendations regarding placement and interventions for the child.

13. Assign a daily task in which the client reads to his/her

initiating or sustaining conversations. (19, 23, 24, 25)

19. Increase the frequency of positive statements about peer group activities and school performance. (21, 22, 24, 25)

20. Decrease the frequency and severity of aggressive acting-out and negative attention-seeking behaviors due to speech/language frustration. (26, 27)

21. Decrease the frequency and severity of dysfluent speech. (28, 29)

22. Comply with a systematic desensitization program to decrease the rate of speech and control stuttering. (28, 29)

23. Verbalize an understanding of how selective mutism is associated with past loss, trauma, or victimization. (30, 31, 32)

24. Verbally identify the dynamics or conflicts in the family system that contribute to selective mutism. (30, 32)

25. Take prescribed medication as directed by the physician. (3, 33)

___. _____
    _____

___. _____
    _____

___. _____
    _____

parents and then retells the story to build his/her vocabulary.

14. Give a directive for the client and his/her family to go on a weekly outing and afterward require the client to share his/her thoughts and feelings about the outing to increase his/her expressive and receptive language abilities.

15. Confront and challenge the parents about placing excessive or unrealistic pressure on the client to "talk right."

16. Assist the parents in developing realistic expectations about the client's speech/language development.

17. Observe parent-child interactions to assess how family communication patterns affect the client's speech/language development.

18. Explore parent-child interactions to determine whether the parents often speak or fill in pauses for the client to protect him/her from feeling anxious or insecure about speech.

19. Encourage the parents to allow the client to take the lead more often in initiating and sustaining conversations.

20. Teach effective communication skills (e.g., active listening, reflecting feelings, "I" statements) in family

therapy sessions to facilitate the client's speech/language development.

21. Assist the client and his/her parents to develop an understanding and acceptance of the limitations surrounding the speech/language disorder.

22. Reinforce the client's goal attainment in speech therapy.

23. Gently confront the client's pattern of withdrawing in social settings to avoid experiencing anxiety about speech problems.

24. Assign the client the task of contributing one comment to classroom discussion each day to increase his/her confidence in speaking before others.

25. Assign the client the task of sharing toys or objects during show-and-tell to increase his/her expressive language abilities.

26. Teach the client positive coping mechanisms (e.g., relaxation techniques, positive self-talk, cognitive reconstructing) to utilize when encountering frustration with speech/language problems.

27. Teach the client self-control strategies (e.g., cognitive reconstructing, positive self-talk, "stop, look, listen, and think") to inhibit the impulse to act out when en-

countering frustration with speech/language problems.

28. Design and implement a systematic desensitization program in which a metronome is introduced and gradually removed to decrease the client's rate of speech and control stuttering.

29. Teach the client effective anxiety reduction techniques (relaxation, positive self-talk, cognitive reconstructing) to decrease the anticipatory anxiety in social settings and control stuttering.

30. Explore the client's background history of loss, trauma, or victimization that contributed to the emergence of selective mutism.

31. Utilize individual play therapy sessions to help the client express his/her feelings surrounding past loss, trauma, or victimization.

32. Assess the family dynamics that contribute to the client's refusal to speak in some situations.

33. Arrange for a medication evaluation if it is determined that an emotional problem and/or ADHD are interfering with speech/language development.

__. _____

_____

—. _____
  _____

—. _____
  _____

DIAGNOSTIC SUGGESTIONS

Axis I: 315.31   Expressive Language Disorder
            315.32   Mixed Receptive–Expressive Language
                      Disorder
            315.39   Phonological Disorder
            307.0   Stuttering
            307.9   Communication Disorder NOS
            313.23   Selective Mutism
            309.21   Separation Anxiety Disorder
            300.23   Social Phobia

            _____   _____

            _____   _____

Axis II: 317   Mild Mental Retardation
            V62.89   Borderline Intellectual Functioning
            799.9   Diagnosis Deferred
            V71.09   No Diagnosis

            _____   _____

            _____   _____

SUICIDAL IDEATION/ATTEMPT

BEHAVIORAL DEFINITIONS

1. Recurrent thoughts of or a preoccupation with death.
2. Recurrent or ongoing suicidal ideation without any plans.
3. Ongoing suicidal ideation with a specific plan.
4. Recent suicide attempt.
5. History of suicide attempts that required professional or family/friend intervention on some level (e.g., inpatient, safe house, outpatient, supervision).
6. Positive family history of depression and/or suicide and a preoccupation with suicidal thoughts.
7. Expression of a bleak, hopeless attitude regarding life, coupled with recent painful life events that support this attitude (e.g., parental divorce, death of a friend or family member, broken close relationship).
8. Social withdrawal, lethargy, and apathy coupled with expressions of wanting to die.
9. Rebellious and self-destructive behavior patterns (e.g., dangerous drug or alcohol abuse, reckless driving, assaultive anger) that indicate a disregard for personal safety and a desperate attempt to escape from emotional distress.

—. _____
   _____
—. _____
   _____
—. _____
   _____

LONG-TERM GOALS

1. Alleviate the suicidal impulses or ideation and return to the highest previous level of daily functioning.
2. Stabilize the suicidal crisis.
3. Place in an appropriate level of care to address the suicidal crisis.
4. Reestablish a sense of hope for the client and his/her life.
5. Terminate the death wish and return to a zestful interest in social activities and relationships.
6. Cease the perilous lifestyle and resolve the emotional conflicts that underlie the suicidal pattern.

—. _____
   _____

—. _____
   _____

—. _____
   _____

SHORT-TERM OBJECTIVES

1. State the strength of the suicidal feelings, the frequency of the thoughts, and the detail of the plans. (1, 2, 3, 11)

2. Report a decrease in the frequency and intensity of the suicidal ideation. (2, 3, 4)

3. Verbalize a promise (as part of a suicide-prevention contract) to contact the therapist or some other emergency helpline if a serious urge toward self-harm arises. (5, 6, 7, 8)

4. Commit to and follow all the stipulations in the suicide contract. (5, 6, 7, 8)

THERAPEUTIC INTERVENTIONS

1. Assess the client's suicidal ideation, taking into account the extent of the ideation, the presence of primary and backup plans, past attempts, and family history. Then make an appropriate intervention or referral.

2. Assess and monitor the client's suicide potential on an ongoing basis.

3. Notify the client's family and significant others of any severe suicidal ideation. Ask them to form a 24-hour suicide watch until the crisis subsides.

5. The parents increase the safety of the home by removing firearms or other lethal weapons from the client's easy access. (1, 3, 9)

6. Cooperate with hospitalization if the suicidal urge becomes uncontrollable. (2, 5, 10, 11)

7. Increase communication between the suicidal client and his/her parents so the client feels attended to and understood. (12, 13, 14, 15)

8. Identify feelings of sadness, anger, and hopelessness related to a conflicted relationship with the parents. (13, 15)

9. The parents verbalize an understanding of the client's feelings of alienation and hopelessness. (12, 15)

10. Take medications as prescribed and report all side effects. (2, 16, 17)

11. Reestablish a consistent eating and sleeping pattern. (16, 17, 18)

12. Verbalize an understanding of the motives for self-destructive behavior patterns. (4, 19, 20, 21)

13. Verbally report and demonstrate an increased sense of hope for him/herself. (4, 14, 22, 23)

14. Identify the positive aspects, relationships, and achievements in his/her life. (22, 23)

4. Explore the sources of emotional pain underlying the client's suicidal ideation and the depth of his/her hopelessness.

5. Elicit a promise from the client that he/she will initiate contact with the therapist or a helpline if the suicidal urge becomes strong and before any self-injurious behavior.

6. Provide the client with an emergency helpline telephone number that is available 24 hours a day.

7. Make a contract with the client, identifying what he/she will and won't do when experiencing suicidal thoughts or impulses.

8. Offer to be available to the client through telephone contact if a life-threatening urge develops.

9. Encourage the parents to remove firearms or other lethal weapons from the client's easy access.

10. Arrange for hospitalization when the client is judged to be harmful to him/herself.

11. Arrange for the client to take the MMPI or BDI and evaluate the results as to the depth of depression.

12. Meet with the parents to assess their understanding of the causes for the client's distress.

15. Disclose the distress caused by broken romantic or social friendships that has led to feelings of abject loneliness and rejection. (24, 25)

16. Identify how his/her previous attempts to solve interpersonal problems have failed, resulting in helplessness. (4, 14, 24)

17. Strengthen the social support network with friends by initiating social contact and participating in social activities with peers. (25, 26, 27)

18. Develop more positive cognitive processing patterns that maintain a realistic and hopeful perspective. (28, 29)

19. Develop and implement a penitence ritual in which the client who survives an incident fatal to others expresses grief for victims and absolves him/herself of responsibility for surviving. (4, 30)

—. _____
   _____

—. _____
   _____

—. _____
   _____

13. Probe the client's feelings of despair related to his/her family relationships.

14. Review with the client previous problem-solving attempts and discuss new alternatives that are available.

15. Hold family therapy sessions to promote communication of the client's feelings of sadness, hurt, and anger.

16. Assess the need for antidepressant medication and arrange for a prescription, if necessary.

17. Monitor the client for the effectiveness of and compliance with prescribed medication.

18. Encourage normal eating and sleeping patterns and monitor compliance.

19. Interpret the client's sadness, wish for death, or dangerous rebellion as an expression of hopelessness and helplessness (a cry for help).

20. Hold play therapy sessions to explore the client's emotional conflicts surrounding him/herself, the family, and friends.

21. Encourage the client to express his/her feelings related to the suicidal behavior in order to clarify them and increase insight into the causes and motives for the behavior.

22. Assist the client in finding positive, hopeful things in his/her life at the present time.

23. Assist the client in developing coping strategies for suicidal ideation (e.g., more physical exercise, less internal focus, increased social involvement, more expression of feelings).

24. Encourage the client to share feelings of grief related to broken close relationships.

25. Encourage the client to reach out to friends and participate in enriching social activities by assigning involvement in one social activity with his/her peers per week. Monitor and process the experience.

26. Use behavioral rehearsal, modeling, and role play to build the client's social skills with his/her peers.

27. Encourage the client to broaden his/her social network by initiating one new social contact per week versus desperately clinging to one or two friends.

28. Assist the client in developing an awareness of the cognitive messages that reinforce hopelessness and helplessness.

29. Identify and confront catastrophizing tendencies in the client's cognitive processing, allowing for a more realistic

perspective of hope in the face of pain.

30. Develop a penitence ritual for the client who is a survivor of an incident fatal to others and implement it with him/her.

___. _____

_____

___. _____

_____

___. _____

_____

DIAGNOSTIC SUGGESTIONS

Axis I:	296.2x	Major Depression, Single Episode
	296.3x	Major Depression, Recurrent
	300.4	Dysthymic Disorder
	296.xx	Bipolar I Disorder
	296.89	Bipolar II Disorder, Depressed
	311	Depressive Disorder NOS
	309.81	Posttraumatic Stress Disorder
	_____	_____
	_____	_____
Axis II:	301.83	Borderline Personality Disorder
	799.9	Diagnosis Deferred
	V71.09	No Diagnosis
	_____	_____
	_____	_____

Appendix A

BIBLIOTHERAPY SUGGESTIONS

Anxiety

Benson, H. (1975). *The Relaxation Response.* New York: William Morrow.

Elkind, D. (1984). *All Grown Up and No Place to Go: Teenagers in Crisis.* New York: Addison-Wesley.

Elkind, D. (1981). *The Hurried Child: Growing Up Too Fast Too Soon.* New York: Addison-Wesley.

McCauley, C. S., and R. Schachter (1988). *When Your Child Is Afraid.* New York: Simon & Schuster.

Moser, Adolph. (1988). *Don't Pop Your Cork on Mondays!* Kansas City, Mo.: Landmark Editions, Inc.

Attention-Deficit/Hyperactivity Disorder

Hallowell, E., and J. Rafey (1994). *Driven to Distraction.* New York: Pantheon.

Ingersoll, B. (1988). *Your Hyperactive Child.* New York: Doubleday.

Parker, H. (1992). *The ADD Hyperactivity Handbook for Schools.* Plantation, Fla.: Impact Publications.

Phelan, T. (1995). *1-2-3 Magic: Training Your Preschoolers and Preteens to Do What You Want.* Glen Ellyn, Ill.: Child Management, Inc.

Quinn, P., and J. Stern (1991). *Putting on the Brakes.* New York: Magination Press.

Shapiro, L. (1993). *Sometimes I Drive My Mom Crazy, But I Know She's Crazy About Me.* King of Prussia, Pa.: Center for Applied Psychology.

Autism/Pervasive Developmental Disorder

Brill, M. (1994). *Keys to Parenting the Child with Autism.* Hauppauge, N.Y.: Barrons.

Rimland, B. (1964). *Infantile Autism.* New York: Appleton Century Crofts.

Siegel, B. (1996). *The World of the Autistic Child.* New York: Oxford.

Simons, J., and S. Olsihi (1987). *The Hidden Child.* Bethesda, Md.: Woodbine House.

Chemical Dependence

Ackerman, R. (1978). *Children of Alcoholics: A Guide for Educators, Therapists and Parents.* Holmes Beach, Fla.: Learning Publications.

Alcoholics Anonymous (1976). *Alcoholics Anonymous: The Big Book.* New York: AA World Service.

Anonymous (1982). *Narcotics Anonymous Big Book.* Van Nuys, Calif.: N.A. World Service. Independence Press.

Bell, T. (1990). *Preventing Adolescent Relapse.* Independence, Mo.: Herald House.

Black, C. (1982). *It Will Never Happen to Me.* Denver: MAC Printing and Publishing.

Bradshaw, J. (1988). *Bradshaw on: The Family.* Pompano Beach, Fla.: Health Communications.

Brown, S. (1985). *Treating the Alcoholic: A Developmental Model of Recovery.* New York: John Wiley & Sons.

Ellis, D. (1986). *Growing Up Stoned.* Pompano Beach, Fla.: Health Communications, Inc.

Woititz, J. G. (1983). *Adult Children of Alcoholics.* Pompano Beach, Fla.: Health Communications.

Conduct Disorder/Delinquency

Canter, L., and P. Canter (1988). *Assertive Discipline for Parents.* New York: HarperCollins.

Katherine, A. (1991). *Boundaries: Where You End and I Begin.* New York: Simon & Schuster.

Kaye, D. (1991). *Family Rules: Raising Responsible Children.* New York: St. Martins.

Phelan, T. (1995). *1-2-3 Magic: Training Your Preschoolers and Preteens to Do What You Want.* Glen Ellyn, Ill.: Child Management, Inc.

Redl, F., and D. Wineman (1951). *Children Who Hate.* New York: Free Press.

Shore, H. (1991). *The Angry Monster.* King of Prussia, Pa.: Center for Applied Psychology.

Wachel, T., D. York, and P. York (1982). *Toughlove.* Garden City, N.J.: Doubleday.

Depression

Black, C. (1979). *My Dad Loves Me, My Dad Has a Disease.* Denver: MAC.

Ingersoll, B., and S. Goldstein (1995). *Lonely, Sad and Angry: A Parent's Guide to Depression in Children and Adolescents.* New York: Doubleday.

Kerns, L. (1993). *Helping Your Depressed Child.* Rocklin, Calif.: Prima.
Moser, A. (1994). *Don't Rant and Rave on Wednesdays!* Kansas City, Mo.: Landmark Editions, Inc.
Sanford, D. (1993). *It Won't Last Forever.* Sisters, Oreg.: Questar Publishers.

Eating Disorder

Fairburn, C. G. (1995). *Overcoming Binge Eating.* New York: Guilford.
Rodin, J. (1992). *Body Traps.* New York: William Morrow.
Siegel, M., J. Brisman, and M. Weinshel (1988). *Surviving an Eating Disorder: Strategies for Families and Friends.* New York: Harper & Row.

Enuresis/Encopresis

Ilg, F., L. Ames, and S. Baker (1981). *Child Behavior: Specific Advice on Problems of Child Behavior.* New York: Harper & Row.
Millman, H., and C. Schaefer (1977). *Therapies for Children: A Handbook of Effective Treatments for Problem Behaviors.* San Francisco: Jossey-Bass.

Fire Setting

Millman, H., and C. Schaefer (1977). *Therapies for Children: A Handbook of Effective Treatments for Problem Behaviors.* San Francisco: Jossey-Bass.

Gender Identity Disorder

Bradley, S., and K. Zucker (1995). *Gender Identity Disorder and Psychosexual Problems in Children and Adolescents.* New York: Guilford.
Silber, S. (1981). *The Male.* New York: C. Scribner's Sons.

Grief/Loss Unresolved

Gardner, R. (1971). *The Boys and Girls Book About Divorce.* New York: Bantam.
Goff, B. (1969). *Where Is Daddy?* Boston: Beacon Press.
Grollman, E. (1967). *Explaining Death to Children.* Boston: Beacon Press.
Grollman, E. (1975). *Talking About Divorce.* Boston: Beacon Press.
Jewett, C. (1982). *Helping Children Cope with Separation and Loss.* Cambridge, Mass.: Harvard University Press.
LeShan, E. (1976). *Learning to Say Good-bye: When a Parent Dies.* New York: MacMillan.

Nystrom, C. (1990). *Emma Says Goodbye.* Batavia, Ill.: Lion Publishing Co.
Rotes, E., ed. (1981). *The Kids' Book of Divorce.* New York: Vintage.

Learning Disorder/Underachievement

Bloom, J. (1990). *Help Me to Help My Child.* Boston: Little, Brown.
Martin, M., and C. Greenwood-Waltman, ed. (1995). *Solve Your Child's School-Related Problems.* New York: HarperCollins.
Millman, H., C. Schaeter, and J. Cohen (1980). *Therapies for School Behavioral Problems.* San Francisco: Jossey-Bass.
Pennington, B. (1991). *Diagnosing Learning Disorders.* New York: Guilford.
Smith, S. (1979). *No Easy Answers.* New York: Bantam Books.

Low Self-Esteem

Briggs, D. (1970). *Your Child's Self-Esteem.* Garden City, N.Y.: Doubleday.
Dobson, J. (1974). *Hide or Seek: How to Build Self-Esteem in Your Child.* Old Tappan, N.J.: F. Revell Co.
Harris, C., R. Bean, and A. Clark (1978). *How to Raise Teenagers' Self-Esteem.* Los Angeles: Price-Stern-Sloan.
Moser, A. (1991). *Don't Feed the Monster on Tuesday!* Kansas City, Mo.: Landmark Editions, Inc.
Sanford, D. (1986). *Don't Look at Me.* Portland, Oreg.: Multnomah Press.
Shapiro, L. (1993). *The Building Blocks of Self-Esteem.* King of Prussia, Pa.: Center for Applied Psychology.

Mania/Hypomania

DePaulo, R., and K. Ablow (1989). *How to Cope with Depression.* New York: McGraw-Hill.
Dumont, L. (1991). *Surviving Adolescence: Helping Your Child Through the Struggle.* New York: Villard Books.

Mental Retardation

Huff, M., and R. Gibby (1958). *The Mentally Retarded Child.* Boston: Allyn and Bacon.
Millman, J., and C. Schaefer. (1977). *Therapies for Children: A Handbook of Effective Treatments for Behaviors.* San Francisco: Jossey-Bass.
Trainer, M. (1991). *Differences in Common.* Rockville, Md.: Woodbine House.

Oppositional Defiant

Bayard, R. T., and J. Bayard (1983). *How to Deal with Your Acting-Up Teen-ager: Practical Self-Help for Desperate Parents.* New York: M. Evans & Co.

Dobson, J. (1978). *The Strong-Willed Child.* Wheaton, Ill.: Tyndale House.

Ginott, H. (1969). *Between Parent and Teen-ager.* New York: MacMillan.

Kaye, K. (1991). *Family Rules: Raising Responsible Children.* New York: St. Martins.

Wachel, T., D. York, and P. York (1982). *Toughlove.* Garden City, N.J.: Doubleday.

Peer/Sibling Conflict

Baruch, D. (1949). *New Ways in Discipline.* New York: MacMillan.

Faber, A., and E. Mazlish (1982). *How to Talk So Kids Will Listen and Listen So Kids Will Talk.* New York: Avon.

Faber, A., and E. Mazlish (1987). *Siblings Without Rivalry.* New York: Norton.

Ginott, H. (1965). *Between Parent and Child.* New York: MacMillan.

Ginott, H. (1969). *Between Parent and Teen-ager.* New York: MacMillan.

Phobia-Panic/Agoraphobia

Brown, J. (1995). *No More Monsters in the Closet.* New York: Prince Paperbacks.

Garber, S., M. Garber, and R. Spitzman (1993). *Monsters Under the Bed and Other Childhood Fears.* New York: Villard.

Wilson, R. (1986). *Don't Panic: Taking Control of Anxiety Attacks.* New York: Harper & Row.

Physical Abuse Victim

James, B. (1989). *Treating Traumatized Children.* New York: Lexington Books.

Miller, Alice. (1984). *For Your Own Good.* New York: Farrar Straus Giroux.

Monahon, Cynthia. (1993). *Children and Trauma: A Parent's Guide to Helping Children Heal.* New York: Lexington Press.

Psychoticism

Dumont, L. (1991). *Surviving Adolescence: Helping Your Child Through the Struggle.* New York: Villard.

Torrey, M. D., and E. Fuller (1988). *Surviving Schizophrenia: A Family Manual.* New York: Harper & Row.

Runaway

Elkind, D. (1984). *All Grown Up and No Place to Go: Teenagers in Crisis.* New York: Addison-Wesley.

Glenn, S., and J. Nelson (1989). *Raising Self-Reliant Children in a Self-Indulgent World.* Rocklin, Calif.: Prima.

Gordon, T. (1970). *Parent Effectiveness Training (P.E.T.).* New York: Wyden Books.

Millman, H., and C. Schaefer (1977). *Therapies for Children: A Handbook of Effective Treatment for Problem Behaviors.* San Francisco: Jossey-Bass.

Wegscheider, S. (1981). *Another Chance: Hope and Health for the Alcoholic Family.* Palo Alto, Calif.: Science and Behavioral Books.

School Refusal

Martin, M., and C. Greenwood-Waltman, ed. (1995). *Solve Your Child's School-Related Problems.* New York: HarperCollins.

Millman, H., and C. Schaefer (1977). *Therapies for Children: A Handbook of Effective Treatments for Problem Behaviors.* San Francisco: Jossey-Bass.

Separation Anxiety

Fraiberg, S. (1959). *The Magic Years.* New York: Scribners.

Ginott, H. (1965). *Between Parent and Child.* New York: MacMillan.

Ingersoll, B., and S. Goldstein (1995). *Lonely, Sad and Angry: A Parent's Guide to Depression in Children and Adolescents.* New York: Doubleday.

Kerns, L. (1993). *Helping Your Depressed Child.* Rocklin, Calif.: Prima.

Kliman, G., and A. Rosenfeld (1980). *Responsible Parenthood.* New York: Holt, Rinehart, and Winston.

Sexual Abuse Perpetrator

Anonymous (1987). *Hope and Recovery, A Twelve Step Guide for Healing from Compulsive Sexual Behavior.* Minneapolis: Comp. Care Publishers.

Bolton, F., L. Morris, and A. MacEachron (1984). *Males at Risk: The Other Side of Sexual Abuse.* Newbury Park, Calif.: Sage Publications.

Carnes, P. (1983). *Out of the Shadows: Understanding Sexual Addiction.* Minneapolis: Comp. Care Publications.

Katherine, A. (1991). *Boundaries: Where You End and I Begin.* New York: Simon & Schuster.

Sanford, D. (1993). *Something Must Be Wrong with Me.* Sisters, Oreg.: Questar Publications.

Sexual Abuse Victim

Carnes, P. (1983). *Out of the Shadows: Understanding Sexual Addictions*. Minneapolis, Minn.: Comp Care Publications.

Colao, F., and T. Hosansky (1987). *Your Children Should Know*. New York: Harper & Row.

Davis, L. (1991). *Allies in Healing*. New York: HarperCollins.

Hagan, K., and J. Case (1988). *When Your Child Has Been Molested*. Lexington, Mass.: Lexington Books.

Hindman, J. (1983). *A Very Touching Book . . . For Little People and for Big People*. Durkee, Oreg.: McClure-Hindman Associates.

Jance, J. (1985). *It's Not Your Fault*. Charlotte, N.C.: Kidsrights.

Katherine, A. (1991). *Boundaries: Where You End and I Begin*. New York: Simon & Schuster.

Sanford, D. (1986). *I Can't Talk About It*. Portland, Oreg.: Multnomah Press.

Sanford, D. (1993). *Something Must Be Wrong with Me*. Sisters, Oreg.: Questar Publishers.

Sleep Disturbance

Ferber, R. (1985). *Solve Your Child's Sleep Problems*. New York: Simon & Schuster.

Ilg, F., L. Ames, S. Baker (1981). *Child Behavior: Specific Advice on Problems of Child Behavior*. New York: Harper & Row.

Social Phobia/Shyness

Martin, M., and C. Greenwood-Waltman, ed. (1995). *Solve Your Child's School-Related Problems*. New York: HarperCollins.

Millman, M., C. Schaefer, and J. Cohen (1980). *Therapies for School Behavioral Problems*. San Francisco: Jossey-Bass.

Zimbardo, P. (1987). *Shyness: What It Is and What to Do About It*. New York: Addison-Wesley.

Speech/Language Disorders

Martin, M., and C. Greenwood-Waltman, ed. (1995). *Solve Your Child's School-Related Problems*. New York: HarperCollins.

Millman, M., C. Schaefer, and J. Cohen (1980). *Therapies for School Behavioral Problems*. San Francisco: Jossey-Bass.

Suicidal Ideation/Attempt

Butler, P. (1991). *Talking to Yourself: Learning the Language of Self-Affirmation.* New York: Perigee.

Dumont, L. (1991). *Surviving Adolescence: Helping Your Child Through the Struggle.* New York: Villard Books.

McCoy, K. (1994). *Understanding Your Teenager's Depression.* New York: Perigee.

Appendix B

INDEX OF DSM-IV CODES ASSOCIATED WITH PRESENTING PROBLEMS

Academic Problem   V62.3
   Learning Disorder/
     Underachievement

Acute Stress Disorder   308.3
   Enuresis/Encopresis
   Physical Abuse Victim
   Sex Abuse Victim

**Adjustment Disorder
With Anxiety**   309.24
   Anxiety
   Runaway

**Adjustment Disorder With
Depressed Mood**   309.0
   Depression
   Grief/Loss Unresolved

**Adjustment Disorder With
Disturbance of Conduct**   309.3
   Fire Setting

**Adjustment Disorder With
Mixed Anxiety and
Depressed Mood**   309.28
   Chemical Dependence

**Adjustment Disorder With
Mixed Disturbance of
Emotions and Conduct**   309.4
   Chemical Dependence
   Fire Setting
   Grief/Loss Unresolved
   Runaway

Alcohol Abuse   305.00
   Chemical Dependence

Alcohol Dependence   303.90
   Chemical Dependence
   Mania/Hypomania

Anorexia Nervosa   307.1
   Eating Disorder

Anxiety Disorder NOS   300.00
   Anxiety
   Social Phobia/Shyness

Asperger's Disorder   299.80
   Autism/Pervasive Developmental
     Disorder
   Mental Retardation

**Attention-Deficit/
Hyperactivity Disorder,
Combined Type   314.01**
   Anxiety
   Attention-Deficit/Hyperactivity
      Disorder
   Learning Disorder/
      Underachievement

**Attention-Deficit/Hyperactivity
Disorder NOS   314.9**
   Attention-Deficit/Hyperactivity
      Disorder
   Conduct Disorder/Delinquency
   Oppositional Defiant
   Peer/Sibling Conflict

**Attention-Deficit/Hyperactivity
Disorder, Predominantly
Inattentive Type   314.00**
   Attention-Deficit/Hyperactivity
      Disorder
   Learning Disorder/
      Underachievement

**Attention-Deficit/
Hyperactivity Disorder,
Predominantly Hyperactive-
Impulsive Type   314.01**
   Attention-Deficit/Hyperactivity
      Disorder
   Conduct Disorder/Delinquency
   Fire Setting
   Low Self-Esteem
   Mania/Hypomania
   Oppositional Defiant
   Peer/Sibling Conflict
   Runaway

Autistic Disorder   299.00
   Autism/Pervasive Developmental
      Disorder
   Oppositional Defiant

Bereavement   V62.82
   Depression
   Grief/Loss Unresolved

Bipolar I Disorder   296.xx
   Attention-Deficit/Hyperactivity
      Disorder
   Depression
   Enuresis/Encopresis
   Mania/Hypomania
   Psychoticism
   Sleep Disturbance
   Suicidal Ideation/Attempt

Bipolar II Disorder   296.89
   Depression
   Mania/Hypomania
   Psychoticism
   Sleep Disturbance
   Suicidal Ideation/Attempt

**Bipolar II Disorder,
Depressed   296.89**
   Suicidal Ideation/Attempt

Bipolar Disorder NOS   296.80
   Mania/Hypomania
   Sleep Disturbance

**Borderline Intellectual
Functioning   V62.89**
   Learning Disorder/
      Underachievement
   Low Self-Esteem
   Mental Retardation
   Speech/Language Disorder

**Borderline Personality
Disorder   310.83**
   Runaway
   Suicidal Ideation/Attempt

Brief Psychotic Disorder   298.8
   Psychoticism

Bulimia Nervosa   307.51
   Eating Disorder

Cannabis Abuse   305.20
   Chemical Dependence

Disorder of Written Expression   315.2
   Learning Disorder/
     Underachievement

Disruptive Behavior Disorder NOS   312.9
   Attention-Deficit/Hyperactivity
     Disorder
   Conduct Disorder/Delinquency
   Oppositional Defiant
   Peer/Sibling Conflict
   Sleep Disturbance

Dissociative Disorder NOS   300.15
   Physical Abuse Victim
   Sexual Abuse Victim

Dysthymic Disorder   300.4
   Chemical Dependence
   Depression
   Eating Disorder
   Enuresis/Encopresis
   Grief/Loss Unresolved
   Learning Disorder/
     Underachievement
   Low Self-Esteem
   Physical Abuse Victim
   Runaway
   School Refusal
   Sleep Disturbance
   Social Phobia/Shyness
   Suicidal Ideation/Attempt

Eating Disorder NOS   307.50
   Eating Disorder

Encopresis With Constipation and Overflow Incontinence   787.6
   Enuresis/Encopresis

Encopresis Without Constipation and Overflow Incontinence   307.7
   Enuresis/Encopresis

Enuresis (Not Due to a General Medical Condition)   307.6
   Enuresis/Encopresis

Exhibitionism   302.4
   Sexual Abuse Perpetrator

Expressive Language Disorder   315.31
   Speech/Language Disorder

Gender Identity Disorder in Adolescents   302.85
   Gender Identity Disorder

Gender Identity Disorder in Children   302.6
   Gender Identity Disorder

Gender Identity Disorder NOS   302.6
   Gender Identity Disorder

Generalized Anxiety Disorder   300.02
   Anxiety
   Low Self-Esteem
   Physical Abuse Victim
   School Refusal
   Separation Anxiety
   Social Phobia/Shyness

Hallucinogen Abuse   305.30
   Chemical Dependence

Hallucinogen Dependence   304.50
   Chemical Dependence

Impulse Control Disorder NOS   312.30
   Fire Setting
   Runaway

Intermittent Explosive Disorder   312.34
   Conduct Disorder/Delinquency

Learning Disorder NOS   315.9
Learning Disorder/
    Underachievement
Peer/Sibling Conflict

**Major Depressive
Disorder   296.xx**
Enuresis/Encopresis
Physical Abuse Victim
School Refusal
Separation Anxiety
Sexual Abuse Victim
Sleep Disturbance
Social Phobia/Shyness

**Major Depressive Disorder,
Recurrent   296.3x**
Depression
Grief/Loss Unresolved
Suicidal Ideation/Attempt

**Major Depressive Disorder,
Recurrent With Psychotic
Features   296.34**
Psychoticism

**Major Depressive
Disorder, Single Episode   296.2x**
Depression
Grief/Loss Unresolved
Suicidal Ideation/Attempt

**Major Depressive Disorder,
Single Episode With
Psychotic Features   296.24**
Psychoticism

Mathematics Disorder   315.1
Learning Disorder/
    Underachievement

**Mental Retardation,
Severity Unspecified   319**
Autism/Pervasive Developmental
    Disorder
Mental Retardation

Mild Mental Retardation   317
Autism/Pervasive Developmental
    Disorder
Learning Disorder/
    Underachievement
Low Self-Esteem
Mental Retardation
Speech/Language Disorder

**Mixed Receptive-Expressive
Language Disorder   315.32**
Speech/Language Disorder

**Moderate Mental
Retardation   318.0**
Mental Retardation

**Neglect of Child
(995.52, Victim)   V61.21**
Low Self-Esteem
Runaway

Nightmare Disorder   307.47
Physical Abuse Victim
Sexual Abuse Victim
Sleep Disturbance

No Diagnosis   V71.09
Anxiety
Attention-Deficit/Hyperactivity
    Disorder
Autism/Pervasive Developmental
    Disorder
Chemical Dependence
Conduct Disorder/Delinquency
Depression
Eating Disorder
Enuresis/Encopresis
Fire Setting
Gender Identity Disorder
Grief/Loss Unresolved
Learning Disorder/
    Underachievement
Low Self-Esteem
Mania/Hypomania
Mental Retardation

Oppositional Defiant
Peer/Sibling Conflict
Phobia-Panic/Agoraphobia
Physical Abuse Victim
Psychoticism
Runaway
School Refusal
Separation Anxiety
Sexual Abuse Perpetrator
Sexual Abuse Victim
Sleep Disturbance
Social Phobia/Shyness
Speech/Language Disorder
Suicidal Ideation/Attempt

**Oppositional Defiant
Disorder   313.81**
Attention-Deficit/Hyperactivity
    Disorder
Chemical Dependence
Conduct Disorder/Delinquency
Peer/Sibling Conflict
Physical Abuse Victim
Runaway

Panic With Agoraphobia   300.21
Phobia-Panic/Agoraphobia

**Panic Without
Agoraphobia   300.22**
Phobia-Panic/Agoraphobia

**Parent-Child Relational
Problem   V61.20**
Conduct Disorder/Delinquency
Runaway

Pedophilia   302.2
Sexual Abuse Perpetrator

**Personality Change Due to
(Axis III Disorder)   310.1**
Depression
Mania/Hypomania
Psychoticism

**Pervasive Developmental
Disorder NOS   299.80**
Autism/Pervasive Developmental
    Disorder
Enuresis/Encopresis

Phonological Disorder   315.39
Speech/Language Disorder

**Physical Abuse of Child
(995.54, Victim)   V61.21**
Low Self-Esteem
Physical Abuse Victim
Runaway

**Posttraumatic Stress
Disorder   309.81**
Enuresis/Encopresis
Physical Abuse Victim
School Refusal
Separation Anxiety
Sexual Abuse Victim
Sleep Disturbance
Social Phobia/Shyness
Suicidal Ideation/Attempt

Primary Hypersomnia   307.44
Sleep Disturbance

Primary Insomnia   307.42
Sleep Disturbance

**Profound Mental
Retardation   318.2**
Mental Retardation

**Reactive Attachment
Disorder of Infancy
or Early Childhood   313.89**
Autism/Pervasive Developmental
    Disorder

Reading Disorder   315.00
Peer/Sibling Conflict

Relational Problem NOS   V62.81
Oppositional Defiant
Peer/Sibling Conflict

Notes

Notes

Notes

Notes

Notes

Notes

Notes

Notes